CARLTON FREDERICKS'
Nutrition Guide

for the Prevention

and Cure of

Common Ailments

and Diseases

Carlton Fredericks, Ph.D.

A FIRESIDE BOOK
Published by Simon and Schuster
New York

A Fireside Book
Published by Simon and Schuster
A Division of Gulf & Western Corporation
Simon & Schuster Building
Rockefeller Center
1230 Avenue of the Americas
New York, New York 10020
FIRESIDE and colophon are registered trademarks of Simon & Schuster.

Designed by *JUDY ALLAN*

Manufactured in the United States of America

Printed and bound by Fairfield Graphics
10 9 8 7 6 5 4 3
Library of Congress Cataloging in Publication Data
Fredericks, Carlton.
    Carlton Fredericks' Nutrition guide for the prevention and cure of common ail-
ments and diseases.

    "A Fireside book."
    Includes bibliographical references and index.
    1. Diet therapy. 2. Vitamin therapy. 3. Minerals in nutrition. I. Title. II. Title:
Nutrition guide for the prevention and cure of common ailments and diseases.
RM217.F73 1982   613.2   82-10705
ISBN: 0-671-44509-X

ACKNOWLEDGMENT

Behind so wide-ranging a book as this, there are many months of bibliographical research, demanding infinite attention to detail and accuracy. One of my former university students, now a medical technician in the field of nutrition, volunteered for that arduous task, greatly easing my responsibilities. I wish to express my gratitude to Inez Sabino.

Behind every successful author, there is likely to be an editor who is the catalyst initiating the chemical reactions that produce a book. My catalyst is Angela Miller, editor-in-chief of Fireside Books, without whose encouragement and enthusiasm this text would have remained unborn.

DEDICATION

To Dr. David Sheinkin—who knew the true meaning of friendship

who was always available to listen to his patients
to befriend his friends
to give guidance and wisdom and love
whatever the problem and whatever the hour

and he in turn was blessed in his relationship with
his beautiful wife and their four children

In his short lifetime he gave so much
to so many

we love you, David

CONTENTS

CONTENTS   **xi**

PROLOGUE

"Nothing Can Be That Effective for So Many Disorders!"

A pioneer in research with DMSO (dimethyl sulfoxide) once remarked that his application for a license to market the drug had been refused because "it was good for too many purposes." Had he confined his claims to the relief of sprained ankles, he remarked bitterly, there would have been no problems with the authorities.

Modern nutrition is in much the same position. The orthodox physician and dietician begin with suspicions of any claims for nutritional therapies not recommended (or not even discussed) in their textbooks. They finish with the ringing declaration that any panacea is suspect, meaning that claims are made for nutrition in too many disorders.

The remarks are seated in something more than unwillingness to accept innovation. They are based on a profound ignorance of the pathways of action through which nutrients operate in health and disease. Consider, for instance, the claims that a single nutritional therapy is helpful or curative in premenstrual syndrome, cystic breast disease, periodontal disease, eczema, arthritis, mental disorders and circulatory diseases. "Snake oil!" is the likely response from the nutritionally unsophisticated. Is it?

The body produces a group of short-lived hormones, the prostaglandins. They are synthesized as they are needed, and disappear when their work is done. This makes them, obviously, difficult to study. One of these is prostaglandin E_1. It is manufactured in the cells from a precursor, dihomogamma linoleic acid. This in turn is manufactured from gamma linoleic acid, and that, in turn, originates with its precursor: linoleic acid. This fatty acid is acquired from food or manufactured from a precursor in vegetable oils: linoleic acid. There the sequence ends: The body can't make linoleic acid to start this progression, and it can't proceed to the third step, gamma linoleic acid, unless there is an adequate supply of other nutrients vital to the process. These include vitamin C, vitamin E, niacinamide, zinc, vitamin B_6, and magnesium. Opposing factors may be present, which will interfere. Even if the nutrients are present in adequate amounts, prostaglandin E_1 will not be formed in adequate quantities in alcoholics, in diabetics who lack insulin, in people who eat excessive amounts of animal (saturated) fat, or in those who ingest too much of the "trans" fats, which are formed in partial hydrogenation of vegetable oils, a technique often employed in everything from margarine to cookies.

The common denominator in the treatment of the disorders I named—alcholism, mental disease, premenstrual syndrome, cystic breast disease, periodontal disease, eczema, arthritis, and circulatory diseases—isn't zinc, magnesium, vitamin B_6, or any of the other nutritional factors. The common denominator is the diverse actions of prostaglandin E_1. While traditional medicine rejects the view of nutrition as a panacea, it finds no difficulty in accepting a prostaglandin deficiency as a factor in a long list of disorders.

No one can understand the complexity of nutrition by studying one facet of it. Nutrients cannot be studied in a vacuum, but must be appraised in terms of their roles in the unbelievably complex chemistry of the body. Nor can the effects of nutritional deficiency be described by statements such as "Vitamin C deficiency causes scurvy." Vitamin C is needed to make the "glue" that binds our cells and tissues together. It is needed to detoxify some of the harmful compounds that find their way into our food supply and bodies. It is a part of the machinery of electron flow in the cells. One can not explain rain in terms merely of "too much moisture in the air," which is the equivalent of "Vitamin C deficiency causes scurvy." Nutrients have many functions other than preventing us from reaching the terminal stage of deficiencies.

Certainly, not all diseases are triggered by the failure of diet to meet our needs; but there is no disease that does not ultimately involve malnutrition, if only at the cellular level.

The Proper Diet—for What and for Whom?

It may occur to you that my emphasis in this text is on individual nutrients or combinations of them, rather than on total diet. There is a very good reason for the omission. I can tailor a diet competently only if I know the indication—the disorder to be addressed, and, even more important, something detailed about the characteristics of the person who will eat that diet.

I can't reduce you with a 1,200-calorie diet ordinarily taking 50 percent of its calories from starch, until I know whether you're one of the very large population who have an unhappy facility for turning carbohydrates into fat rather than energy. For them, only a low-carbohydrate diet will do, and calories are a secondary consideration.

I can't put you on a high-protein diet for hypoglycemia, unless I warn you that carbohydrate tolerances differ from person to person and that some hypoglycemics need more than others, and some less.

If you are a schizophrenic or you are feeding an autistic child, I have no right to frame a diet until allergies are checked. The protein innocuous and helpful to one person may create hallucinations in another who is schizophrenic, or more head-banging and rocking in an autistic child.

This should come as no revelation. I've already expressed my scientific distaste for the "one-note" players in the field of nutrition, who have a single dietary approach to all mankind and all ills.

The doctrine goes so far that I can't even be safe in assuming that the dietary habits of a seventy-year-old must represent a success story and require no change. Does one assume that the octane need of a car in its eighth year is identical with that of its first?

The omission of dietary imperatives protects you. It honors individual differences, and, on the basis of long experience, I can tell you that our differences, nutritionally, are greater than our similarities.

INTRODUCTION

This book is dedicated to a singular biochemical event in the universe: you. It is an antidote for the illusions (and harm) created by those who promise a uniform response to uniform nutrition by a nonuniform public. It replies to the "one-note" players in the nutrition orchestra—those who believe that a single type of diet and a list of uniform vitamin and mineral requirements are the sole path to well-being for *everybody.* Exponents of that kind of rigid dogma range from the American Heart Association to Nathan Pritikin, and their philosophy recalls John Dewey's remark that Americans prefer to *know* rather than to *think,* for certainty is secure, and speculation filled with anxiety.

When nutritional treatment helps the suffering, my joy is tinged with a note of regret, for such victories are often monuments to lost opportunities for prevention. The arthritic who responds to a nutritional therapy might have avoided the disease by intelligent selection of menus. The schizophrenic whose sanity is restored with nutrient treatment might never have been psychotic if his prior nutrition had been good enough to help him better to resist stress. The vitamin C and gamma linoleic acid that helped to tighten someone's loose teeth could have been applied earlier for prevention. Another person's cystic mastitis might never have arisen to torture her if the vitamin E that helped her to recover had been better supplied by her diet—and it would have been, if she had chosen whole grains instead of white flour and other caricatures of cereal and grain foods. The vitamin B_6, zinc, lecithin, folic acid, and linoleic acid that sometimes slow down or even reverse atherosclerosis (hardening of the arteries) obviously could have been preventively supplied by the patient's previous food and supplement selections. Herein lies one of the great differences between orthomolecular nutrition and drug-oriented treatment: You can't take digitalis today to prevent the heart attack of tomorrow.

There are, of course, exceptions to the generalization that nutrition ordinarily prevents what it cures. If a massive dose of vitamin C is administered intravenously to bring your hepatitis under control—which it will, in half the time required by orthodox care—this doesn't mean that an extra glass of orange juice daily would have warded off the infection. Yet there *is* a use of the vitamin in preventing serum hepatitis, for patients treated with it prior to receiving blood transfusions are *much* less likely to suffer with this frequent infection. And the fact that we know this is so, from studies in both the United States and Japan, has, infuriatingly, had no impact on medical practices here, for tens of thousands of critically ill or injured patients continue to receive transfusions, minus the vitamin protection, and a predictable percentage of them do develop serum hepatitis, which, as you probably know, is not a minor hazard. That is an example of the cultural lag, the gap between findings and their acceptance and application for the benefit of suffering humanity.

As the classic example of cultural lag, you have doubtless heard of the struggle of the nineteenth-century Hungarian physician Ignaz Semmelweiss, who could not persuade his colleagues that they must not go from autopsies to delivering babies without washing their hands. Many of you will recall that his peers jeered at him, destroyed his medical career, and ultimately drove him insane, but few know that he used his suicide in a last, despairing effort to convince doctors that bacteria from dead bodies, conveyed to women in labor, were responsible for deadly childbirth fever. He killed himself by plunging a scalpel, previously used in an autopsy, into his own hand; he died because of the infection.

And if you want a demonstration that cultural lag is real, consider that in 1981 a major medical journal, The *New England Journal of Medicine,* scolded physicians for going from one patient to another without washing their hands. One of my physician friends, Dr. William Kaufman, whose discoveries in vitamin therapy for arthritis were buried in the same cultural chasm, ironically remarked that it is perhaps fortunate that Semmelweiss's battle didn't take place in this enlightened age, for his peers would have insisted that the research wasn't "double blind." The term is shorthand for a testing technique designed to rule out any benefits that actually derive from the physician's expectations and the patient's faith and hope; in other words, from the power of suggestion. One group of patients receives the actual treatment; the other, unknowingly, receive a sham treatment, or placebo, which they believe to be real. Not only are the subjects unaware of the group they're in, but the researchers themselves do not know, until the experiment is over. On occasion, a cross-over technique embellishes the double-blind test. In this, after the first trial, the two groups change places (unknowingly), and those who were receiving the actual medication now take the inactive placebo, and vice versa. To my mind, double-blind studies set impossible goals. It is often difficult, if not impossible, to evaluate subjective improvements from nutritional therapy, and yet many responses to such treatment must be gauged by how the patient feels and functions. For this reason, much nutrition research is not double blind.

Let me give you an idea of the frivolity of the rejection of nutrition research on the grounds that it isn't double blind. Let us say that I suspect that your arthritis began with a sensitivity to toxic chemicals in potato, tomato, eggplant, peppers, and tobacco. (This isn't hypothetical. You'll find it explained in the section on arthritis. Up to 70 percent of arthritics tested have such sensitivity.) Suppose I order these foods withdrawn from your diet, with the result that three or four months later, you have increased mobility of your joints and reduced swelling, tenderness, and pain. Does this prove my case to my satisfaction? Not quite: I'll ask you to eat the tabooed foods for a few days, and observe what happens. It turns out that your joints again trouble you, and swelling and tenderness return. Does this satisfy the orthodoxy in medicine and nutrition? No. It isn't double blind. I must repeat the research and give you the offending chemicals in capsule form, and give others a placebo capsule. Otherwise, I've not ruled out the possibility that my charming personality and your faith in what I do may have been the healing agent. Net result: My treatment won't be used. This is in spite of the fact that there is a new case of arthritis every thirty seconds or so, and that the drugs prescribed for it have side reactions often worse than the disease. I might add that the Arthritis Foundation is not likely to accept my results even when the double-blind technique is used because of a dogged insistence that diet has nothing to do with the disease.

That is cruel enough, but there is another question. What if you are a physician who knows in advance, as I do, that what you are doing for the patient with diet helps 70 percent of the victims of arthritis? Will you, in the name of science, exploit the next sufferer by giving him a placebo? Another version of that cruelty appears in the cross-over technique previously mentioned. Let's apply it to multiple sclerosis. In this book is a description of a therapy I know to be helpful in about 25 percent of the cases. Should I use the double blind, which means tricking these grievously sick people by giving them an inactive "treatment," and then compound the cruelty by withdrawing the actual therapy from the first group, putting them on the placebo, and therby depriving some of them of the benefits they've already enjoyed?

Don't treat these notes as academic. For one thing, they explain why so much of the information in this text will be new to you and your practitioner. They also explain my prophecy that today's medicine will be severely criticized in the centuries to come—not for the ignorance it represents, which is understandable, but for its pretensions. As an example, consider that a few years ago, New Jersey researchers studied the effectiveness of folic acid, a B complex vitamin, in preventing congenital spinal deformities—the neural tube defects that cripple the newborn and often sentence them to an early death. These researchers reported the vitamin effective for a significant percentage of the pregnant women studied. Nonetheless, British physicians *recently* repeated the study, and though they knew in advance that the treatment is effective in preventing these abnormalities, and although they were aware that mothers who have borne one such crippled child are at greater risk of bearing another one, they nonetheless used such women for a double-blind test. In the group given the inactive pills, the rate of such births was significantly higher; the babies of women treated with folic acid were largely protected by the vitamin. Thus, in the name of science, defective babies were brought into the world. The mothers, the researchers said piously, gave "informed consent" to the procedure. Was it justified? Were there any grounds for belief that the power of suggestion, rather than folic acid, might have corrected whatever deficiency caused the spinal deformities?

Physicians who read this book may respond, when you ask for help in applying its suggestions, that the research behind my data is not acceptable—that it's based largely on the anecdotal. You might remind them that much of their own education was based on untested medical dogma or experience, often minus *any* research, controlled or uncontrolled. They prescribed aspirin for fifty years before any of its actions—some of them distinctly undesirable—were understood. They performed the "radical mastectomy" for ninety years before they tested it against a simple mastectomy or lumpectomy, plus radiation, to discover that the more drastic operation, with its crippling and deforming effects, was no more effective. They administered estrogen to menopausal women for a half-century, though they had only one "controlled" research project to back its use, and that one showed the placebo to be as effective as the hormone. Estrogen, not at all incidentally, causes five species of animals to develop eleven types of cancer.

Why, then, the caution with nutrients that in appropriate (and effective) doses are harmless? Why the demand to eliminate the placebo effect? And if nutrition, as some cynics insist, derives half of its beneficial actions from a placebo effect, can you think of a placebo that is as effective and as free of side reactions?

It is my goal in this book to fill what I perceive as a gap between the nutritional research that is buried in journals or books gathering dust in the scientific libraries, and an awareness of it by the public. There are nutritional treatments that are the results of unpublished research, including some of my own, which could be helpful to many. I don't want that research to remain inaccessible.

It is true that we have had a cascade of books on nutrition in health and disease, including some ten of my own, but primarily they are devoted to single topics, such as arthritis, hypoglycemia, and diabetes. It appeared to me that no one had effectively gathered in one text all the available information on such therapies and, more important, the lessons they teach in possible prevention, and that is what I have done in this book. This book is for the women who do not realize that nutritional therapies offer an alternative to hysterectomies for uterine fibroid tumors, operations performed at the rate of more than 200,000 yearly. This book is for the depressed and suicidal patients who aren't likely to learn that there is nutritional treatment that may free them from tranquilizers, shock therapy, and years on the psychoanalytic couch. This book is for parents of autistic children who are seldom aware that foods, drugs, and chemicals involved in cerebral allergy may be responsible for a good part of the symptoms. This book is for the victims of regional ileitis (Crohn's disease) who are unaware that simple, harmless nutritional treatment may offer help in mitigating symptoms and, indeed, in escaping surgery. Those who suffer from the devastating effects of chemotherapy and irradiation for cancer rarely, if ever, are aware that those side reactions can be lessened or even banished if the science of nutrition is properly applied. The symptoms of hypoglycemia (low blood sugar) often are "treated" with mind-bending drugs, years of psychiatric therapy, and even, heaven help the patient, shock therapy. This book is for them and others who suffer from a myriad of disorders that are responsive to treatment with diet and nutrients. It is important that you realize that it wasn't written to equip you to be your own doctor, for the saying goes that the self-medicated have a fool for a doctor and another for a patient. It isn't that nutrient and dietary therapies are inherently dangerous, though the defenders of drugs may make it appear so, for nutrients are infinitely safer than drugs.

But there is a risk with self-medication with nutrients. Let me tell you why.

1. Mistaken diagnosis. You may not be treating what you think you are. Your symptoms, for instance, may suggest a stomach ulcer, but nutritional therapy doesn't help, because you may have all the symptoms, but you don't have an ulcer. What you have, in this hypothetical case, is TMJ dysfunction, resulting from an improper alignment of the teeth, throwing the jaw out of alignment. This can result in symptoms ranging from hearing loss to pain in the face *and* all the symptoms of gastric ulcer. The condition can be remedied by dentists who specialize in treating it, but vitamin and diet therapy for ulcer, obviously, will do nothing for it. Low blood sugar, I might mention, can also cause all the digestive symptoms of an ulcer. Since the diet for both conditions is often identical, you may rid yourself of an imaginary ulcer by accidentally treating hypoglycemia. The risk here is in the nature of both disorders: the tendency to gastric ulcer, like the tendency to hypoglycemia, is rarely cured. It is controlled.

2. Missed diagnosis. You may be treating what you think you are, but you may have another underlying disorder, undetected and thereby untreated. An example is vitiligo, described as a harmless but cosmetically distressing depigmentation of the skin, cause unknown. Nutrition articles tell you that PABA, a B complex factor, occasionally recolors the depigmented areas. But vitiligo may be a warning that the hydrochloric acid level in your stomach is too low, which could be a prelude to pernicious anemia—for which PABA is ineffective.

3. Overlooked problems with allergy or intolerance. There is nothing on the face of the earth—or for that matter, in our polluted air—to which someone, somewhere, is not allergic. It is possible to be allergic to vitamins, minerals, protein foods, spices, or even the binders and fillers used in nutritional supplements and drugs. As an example, consider the person violently allergic to corn, who reacts adversely to vitamin C tablets for the reason that most ascorbic acid

is derived from corn. For such an individual, the vitamin must be synthesized from another base—sago palm. But how many laymen are aware that such a form of vitamic C is available? The self-medicator must be sensitively aware of his or her allergies and intolerances.

4. Incorrect dosage. Recognizing the need to lower or raise dosage is a problem for the medical nutritionist, and it is obviously a greater difficulty for the untrained. As an example, suppose you discover that your constant depression and suicidal thoughts may be caused by excessive copper intake, possibly originating with a soft-water supply conducted through copper piping. You learn that zinc is used to lower blood copper levels, but when you take a zinc supplement, you actually feel more depressed. Discouraged, you throw out the zinc tablets. The medical nutritionist could have told you that zinc does bring down blood copper levels, but if the amount of copper in the body is excessive, it will first be moved from the tissues where it has been stored to the blood, to replace its falling levels there. This means that zinc may temporarily *raise* blood copper levels. The remedy is clear to the nturitionally sophisticated: you lower the dose of zinc to slow up the process. The layman might also fail to recognize that your dose is inadequate. You've read that the body can utilize only a microgram or so of vitamin B_{12} daily, and you're taking 500 micrograms because you hope it will help your cold sores or shingles (herpes infections). No response, and for a very good reason. Vitamin B_{12} is absorbed so poorly that injections are almost always preferred by physicians. There *is* an exception: the vitamin is available in tablets to be dissolved under the tongue, allowing quick and efficient absorption. If you don't know about these "linguets" nor the reason they are a preferred way of taking the vitamin, you lose the opportunity to help yourself.

In addition, much is likely to be lost if you try to diagnose and treat yourself. You have read that vitamin B_6 and the vitamin B complex sometimes relieve premenstrual symptoms and shorten the menstrual period. They do, if the B complex supplement is properly formulated for those purposes. Most of them on the market are not. But for the majority of women, there is more to offer than a lessening of menstrual discomfort. With supplements and improved nutrition, what may be possible is prevention of cystic breast disease, uterine fibroid tumors, and a common type of breast cancer. To take full advantage of nutrition as a weapon against these common disorders, supplements alone are not enough. If the woman is allergic, the removal of allergenic foods from the diet is also helpful. If she is a user of coffee, tea, chocolate, cocoa, and other sources of caffeine, she must stop. Finally, her sugar intake must be drastically lowered, and her protein and vitamin E level raised to meet her needs. A number of disorders women believe to be the inevitable price of having been born female and being able to conceive may be corrected by diet and supplements.

So it is that I strongly advise against self-medication. This may seem contradictory when you read the text, for in places I supply both the supplementary levels of nutrient intake and the therapeutic *range;* but you will realize that I intend this book to guide not only the layman interested in prevention, but also the professional who seeks the protocols for nutritional therapies. It may be heresy to address a book both to the public and the professions, but experience has taught me that it can be done, for not only has my book on hypoglycemia for the general public been used as a guide by many practitioners, but in turn they have made it mandatory reading for appropriate patients.

In the past, the medical professions have not looked kindly upon nutritionists, lay or medical, and they have reserved special hostility for nonmedical practitioners such as myself. But this antagonism is waning, however slowly, if I am to judge from recent letters from physicians, dentists, and psychiatrists. Their questions tell the story:

M.D.: "My wife is about to undergo cobalt therapy for a neoplasm in her larynx. What are the nutritional antioxidants that may offset the side effects?"

D.D.S.: "I heard your interview on the prostaglandins when you talked with Dr. David Horrobin. Would the gamma linoleic acid in evening primrose oil stimulate enough prostaglandin synthesis to make it useful in treating periodontal disease?"

M.D. (surgeon): "I am interested in the nutritional treatment of Down's syndrome. Can you supply the nutritional therapy, or guide me to the literature on the subject?"

M.D. (allergist): "I have frankly been skeptical about food allergy and particularly about cerebral allergy. Please send me a bibliography and, if possible, the name of a qualified practitioner in those areas, whose work I might observe. Are you saying that cerebral allergy literally can cause psychosis?" (Answer: yes.)

M.D. (psychiatrist): "Why is it advisable to prescribe magnesium when treating an autistic child with pyridoxine [vitamin B$_6$]?" (Answer: If you don't, the results will be sensitivity to noise, irritability, and bed-wetting.)

M.D. (medical nutritionist): "Prostate trouble stymies me. I think of zinc and stop there. There must be more one can do." (Answer: Yes. Use vitamin B$_6$ to improve absorption of zinc; vitamin C for its diuretic effect; vitamin E and vegetable oil to improve circulation.)

M.D. (pediatrician): "Why is there such a wide range of responses of hyperactive children to a diet free of additives, dyes, etc.?" (Answer: There are actually four different types of brain neurotransmitter disturbances in these children. Each responds differently.)

It becomes obvious that the professions are now interested in nutrition.

This book discusses the application of nutrition to a wide variety of disorders, from relatively rare ones, like Sjögren's syndrome and brain damage, to common ones like senility and strokes. Where I have reason to believe that the rationale for the therapy will not be familiar to the average medical practitioner, I supply it. I do not usually supply therapeutic doses, but professionals are welcome to write to me, in care of my publisher, for such information. For the general public, dosages recommended are in terms of preventive nutrition. I should also note that there is usually no relationship between these preventive levels and Recommended Dietary Allowances. Experience tells me that the RDAs are too low for many of us, but thanks to the research of Dr. Roger Willaims, I also know that the dietary allowances will exactly fit the needs of only 33 people in every 1,000. The others have requirements that, as happens with all averages, will fall above and below the average. For the same reason, I make no generalizations about the kind of diet you should be eating. I believe that such generalizations, like the RDAs, make about as much sense as a proposal to make dentures or bras in one size for manufacturing economy.

There are few quick miracle cures in nutrition. It took years for you to eat your way into trouble; improvement with corrected diet requires concentrated nutrition, plus a seasoning of weeks, months, or even years for full recovery. Moreover, the body remembers insults: It may have taken twenty years for you to slide into the pit of ill health based on nutritional imbalances and deficiencies, but after you're rescued you will find it will take only months of renewed dietary sinning to bring the symptoms back.

A lesson was once taught to me by a woman who, learning my identity, gasped: "Dr. Fredericks! *You* wear glasses?" I responded by noting that my mother, when bearing me, refused to take any advice from me. The point is that you must not expect supernutrition to make you a superhuman being. All we can hope for is your reaching your full potential; few people do. No diet changes a mouse into an elephant, but good nutrition can help the mouse to live longer, resist disease, respond better when medication is needed, and function at a higher level.

I write of mice, but I speak to men and women.

Carlton Fredericks, Ph.D., F.R.S.H., F.I.A.P.M.
New City, New York
1982

ACNE

Until one or two years ago, many dermatologists were dosing acne patients with antibiotics, sometimes for periods of years. With equal conviction, they now assert that hormonal imbalance is responsible for this skin disease, justifying glandular therapy. Although they find it currently fashionable to deny that diet plays any part in acne, I remember a statement made by a physician, a diplomate in dermatology, who for years was my associate in research in nutrition. "A rise in blood glucose [sugar]," he said, "is multiplied by five when it reaches the skin." His point: Sugar-saturated skin is a happy hunting ground for bacteria. Diabetics will have learned to agree. That takes us back to the acne diet of decades ago: It is important to reduce the intake of sugar. Unfortunately, sealing the sugar bowl doesn't accomplish that, for much of our sugar intake is concealed in foods. Ketchup contains 20 percent sugar, Shake 'n Bake is 50 percent sugar, canned green peas are sugared, a doughnut contains five teaspoonfuls and a portion of apple pie twelve teaspoonfuls; there is even sugar in the antacid tablet you take for the indigestion fanned by too much sugar.

Several nutrients have proved beneficial in acne. These include vitamin A, 5,000 to 10,000 units daily; high-potency vitamin B complex; vitamin B_6, 10 mg. daily; lecithin, one to two tablespoons of granules daily; and zinc gluconate or a chelated form, 15 to 30 mg. daily. The physician may considerably increase these levels.

ALLERGIES

When allergies have been clearly identified and your biochemistry cooperates enough not to develop new allergies and lose old ones at an unpredictable rate, there are aids in nutrition that are comparatively simple and often quite effective. I have seen hay fever relieved (and even its symptoms eliminated) by the routine use of a timed-release vitamin C supplement, 500 mg., taken at intervals, two or three times daily. Some hay fever sufferers need the impact of larger doses, not timed-release, taken every four or five hours, so that higher blood levels of the vitamin, which is an antihistamine, can be achieved. Others do not respond to vitamin C alone, but may get relief with the addition of a few hundred milligrams of vitamin B_6 to each dose of vitamin C. This treatment does not cure allergy, but does provide relief—when it works, which it doesn't for everyone who uses it.

The combination of vitamins B_6 and C has proved unexpectedly effective in some cases of cerebral allergy (also known as maladaptive reaction) where the symptoms primarily affect mood, emotions, thinking, and perceptions of reality. Unexpected and gratefully received responses sometimes come with vitamin E in hay fever; with vitamin C and bioflavonoids in allergic sinusitis, postnasal drip, and frequent colds. Allergic asthma sometimes responds to vitamin B_{12}, both by injection and with the use of sublingual lozenges.

Generally, though, the first problem is not treatment but identification of allergies. Many sufferers are not aware that allergy is their problem. Over and over, I hear people say they have no allergies—their only problem is frequent colds. They never read the statement made by a pioneering allergist, Arthur F. Coca: "We don't catch colds—we *eat* them." In determining whether your problem is allergy, some of the responsibility falls squarely on *you*. More can be done than the conventional scratch and patch tests of the orthodox allergist. Moreover, his examination will be confined in the straightjacket of the allergy orthodoxy, for their conventional testing methods do not identify food allergy, and indeed, and unbelievably, the official position is that food allergy is simply too "iffy" and may not even exist. That's because it often does not reflect the IgE (immunogobulin E) reaction which is their definition of an allergic reaction. That is small comfort to the person who gets headaches from chocolate, colds from milk, indigestion from scallops, and intense irritability from shrimp. To bypass this philosophical and medical obstacle, I propose to teach you how to identify allergies at home, with which I'll couple some of the examinations performed by allergists who have escaped the straightjacket of the establishment.

You begin by keeping a double-entry diary. On one side of the page, list everything you eat—and the times of eating. On the other side of the page, list any symptoms you have developed—and the time at which they did. Do not confine the entries to food and beverages, though. List any chemicals to which you were exposed, such as insecticide sprayed in your areas, or heavy smoke from burning leaves, or the spray of a fabric softener. List any medication you took, which might range from mouthwash or toothpaste to a headache tablet or your vitamin supplement. Always record the time you took them; always record symptoms and the time they occurred.

Over a period of weeks—and it often takes that long—you may begin to see a pattern emerging. You ate a certain food three times, and on all those occasions—an hour or a few hours later—your nose was stuffy, or you had a headache, or your vision blurred. Two warnings: First, the reaction sometimes may take a day or even longer, complicating the task of establishing the relationship between insult and symptom. Second, and very important, never forget that the foods and drinks you *crave* are very often the offenders, and these entries in the diary must be carefully matched against any symptoms that follow. Conversely, making the matter more complicated, there may be symptoms when you *stop* consuming a favorite food or beverage. If that is puzzling, consider this type of allergy as leading to addiction. Like a drug addict, you crave the food or drink because (a) taking it makes you feel better and (b) not taking it makes you feel terrible. You may not recognize these effects, but allergic addiction is a very real source of some people's troubles.

There is an added device to give you a cross-check on what you learn from the food-symptom diary. Before you leave your bed in the morning, take your pulse for one full minute. Take it again before you eat. Eat *one* food in your usual portion. Forty minutes later, take your pulse again. If it has risen more than eighteen beats, or, whatever the rise, gone over eighty-four beats per minute, there is a strong probability that you are allergic to that food. If the food was innocent, you can repeat it after your pulse has returned to your normal level, and add a second food for the next test. This method may seem slow and cumbersome, but it has a high degree of reliability, and allows you to go back to a full diet, minus the foods and drinks to which you prove sensitive, in a reasonably short time.

There is another method that can be used at home to identify allergies, though I prefer that it be applied by an expert. Chiropractors, one of whom, Dr. George Goodheart, discovered this technique, often have specialized training in kinesiology. This method is based on the idea that certain muscles will be weakened when you are exposed to a food or beverage (or, for that matter, medication, vitamins, or other substances) to which you are allergic. In the oversimplified form in which the test can be tried at home, you extend your arm to the side, parallel with the floor. A partner tests the springiness of the muscles, by gently tugging with one finger, at your wrist area. In other words, he will act as if gently trying to bring your arm down to your side. It is not a test of strength—just one of muscle tone. You now place a food (premoistened) or beverage under your tongue, wait a few minutes, and repeat the arm test. If you find that your muscles noticeably weaken, this is regarded as a positive sign of allergy. It sounds like witchcraft, but after being trained in the technique, I can tell you that it's remarkably (if inexplicably) effective. I might add that the trained kinesiologist will not rely on a test of just one muscle to make a diagnosis.

Another self-care program for the allergic starts with a forty-eight-hour fast, to detoxify the body. Twelve foods are listed for the first three days of testing, and only one of these is eaten at each of four meals per day. Only pure sweet butter and sea salt are allowed as condiments. In the next two days, the fourth and fifth, meals consist of combinations of eight small portions of the twelve foods, not including, of course, any to which you have had an abnormal response. For the next three days, you test four more new foods each day. This adds up to another twelve foods that can be combined for the next test meals combining eight foods. A diary is kept of both foods and symptoms. Symptoms may be mild or severe, but in most instances they are readily detectable by anyone who is striving for a modest degree of self-appraisal. Remember that the symptom doesn't have to be hives, itching, or asthma. It can be a headache or a feeling of depression or anxiety without justification in the life situation; even sleepiness may be a revealing symptom. In severe allergy, there may be an eruption of full-blown symptoms, such as I discuss in the arthritis section of this book, where pain, stiffness, and swelling may be the price for exposure to an allergen.

As technicians sometimes say, there is a "quick and dirty" way of shortening at-home testing. It calls for *total* removal of a food from the diet for five days. Usually, this makes the body hypersensitive to that food, so that taking a normal portion of it for lunch, on the fifth day, may trigger an acute reaction that, under these circumstances, becomes clear and unmistakable. This result is based on the fact that regular consumption of a food to which you are allergic masks the symptoms by invoking the body's defenses. When the food is withdrawn, so are the defenses, and a renewed insult—eating the food—will catch the body off guard.

What you have just read partially justifies a strange observation. A minute does of an offending food sometimes can cancel allergic symptoms. Thus the person who has developed a headache from eating chocolate may eliminate it by swallowing a half-glass of water containing two, three, or four drops of chocolate syrup. Establishing exactly the right amount, obviously, is tricky, but it will be astonishingly small. In alcoholism of the type based on allergy, a few drops of an alcoholic beverage, the addict's favorite, in a glass of water may for many hours eliminate the craving. If you pause to think about this, is it not a scientific version of the doctrine of "the hair of the dog that bit you"?

In place of the scratch and patch tests, the modern allergist may use the same technique used in the kinesiological method, without the muscle testing. He will rely on the subjective reactions of the patient under whose tongue he has placed a solution of a food, chemical, drug, vitamin, or whatever. Usually, the patient doesn't know what is being tested—a "blind" procedure that pleases those who place stress upon the factor of suggestion.

Injections are used by some allergists; others use the RAST test, which is costly, and only about 30 percent accurate, but sometimes useful. Still others use the Rinkel method, which not only has the virtue of establishing sensitivity to the food, but also gives information for a "neutralizing" level of dosage. This is analogous to the chocolate-syrup-in-water technique discussed above.

Sometimes, the test—of whatever type—leads to conclusions that create large problems. People who are allergic to hydrocarbons may have to dispose of plastic tiling in their homes, or get rid of gas stoves with pilot lights. When the symptoms are distressing enough, most patients are compelled to comply. What else do you do when your gas furnace has given you a constant depression on which you've vainly spent a fortune with psychoanalysis and prescriptions for antidepressants?

In extremely severe cases of allergy, where the unfortunates have become prisoners of the disorder, afraid to eat in a restaurant or unable to go to a theater (it may have been sprayed with a deodorant to which they are sensitive), there are now facilities where the patient can be tested. He is sealed into an environment free from the chemicals, insecticide residues, lead, and other contaminants of our world. Air is filtered; water is distilled. After a prolonged fast—never to be attempted without constant medical supervision—the bioecological allergist will test for allergy or intolerance to everything conceivable—foods, drugs, cosmetics, preservatives, food additives, mold, fungi, yeast spores, hydrocarbons, fabrics—and the patient may, sometimes, have to strictly control his environment thereafter.

There *are* occasional reports that doses of a single nutrient, or use of a hypoglycemia diet (see pages 104–105), where appropriate, have banished allergy completely. This is rare with single nutrients, but does occur with vitamins B_{12}, B_6, E, and C and bioflavonoids. It is quite common, though, for a person with low blood sugar to have allergies, and the control of the low blood sugar to eliminate the allergic tendency, or at least make it controllable. Another therapy, long ago reported in the *Annals of Allergy*, an orthodox journal, recorded the disappearance of allergies in patients sensitive to a long list of foods, who were treated with predigested protein and the vitamin B complex. Here the problem may be dual: finding a predigested protein, necessary because the predigestion minimizes the chance of an allergic reaction to the concentrate; and making sure that the person is not allergic to the B vitamins or to the natural B complex base (liver, yeast, etc.) usually incorporated with them.

Still another device helpful for those with multiple food allergies is the four-day rotation diet. As the name implies, this is a menu plan that avoids the repetition of any one food more often than once every four days. The time lapse makes it less likely that one will become sensitized. In the Appendix under Reference Reading, you will find texts listed detailing such diets. One word of caution: A four-day rotation may not be sufficient if you are seriously intolerant of a certain food; the interval will have to be lengthened. You do need guidance in setting up your menus for rotation, if you are to preserve good nutrition and retain some enjoyment in eating.

From decades of observing allergic people, I can tell you that stress is a large part of the problem. So is poor nutrition, for dietary deficiencies can interfere with enzyme systems, making it impossible for your body to metabolize some of the essential chemicals involved in the healthy running of your body.

There is a champion athlete who brings buffalo steaks to his sports events, for this is the only meat he can eat without allergic reactions. There is a girl who could attend college only when she found one where smoking was forbidden. There are people who can't sleep under sheets made of synthetic fibers. There are those whose homes must be heated electrically at today's fantastic prices, because of the deep depressions they develop when exposed to combustion products of gas furnaces. They have solved their problems, at least partially; yours can be solved, too, and you have an advantage, if your physician can teach you how to achieve the best possible nutrition. In the Appendix, you are referred to a society of bioecological allergists. If your problem is severe, a consultation would be a good investment.

THE ANTI-AGING ANTIOXIDANTS IN NUTRITION

Readers and radio listeners often ask about the "secret" of my freedom, at the age of seventy-two, from the wrinkles and the gray hair "normal" at that age. Heredity isn't the explanation, nor yet freedom from stress, for the males in my family aged rapidly and died relatively young; and no one serving the public is free of stress.

Part of the explanation, other than eating a good (not perfect) diet for many decades is found in my generous intake of antioxidant nutrients. "Antioxidant" means "anti-oxygen," which must puzzle the layman, who thinks of oxygen as needed and friendly. When you see iron rusting, though, you are reminded that oxygen can be destructive, if not under control. The destructive role of oxygen in the body is analogous to its effect on oils and fats, which become rancid. This explains the use of preservatives in such foods. Preventing "rancidity" in the cells demands a rich supply of nutritional preservatives. These include Vitamin C, Vitamin E, selenium, sulfur-containing amino acids, superoxide dismutase, and lecithin. Supplements and foods supplying these factors are, of course, available. Only the sulfur-containing amino acids will pose a problem for the uninitiated. Actually, they are richly supplied by eggs and liver. This may explain why, despite the low-cholesterol fad, egg-eaters outlive non-egg-eaters by a significant margin. Vitamin E is not a fully effective antioxidant if taken in the form of alpha tocopherol. The antioxidant action of this vitamin is much higher in the beta, gamma, and delta forms. One buys this by asking for "mixed tocopherols," rather than for alpha tocopherol alone, though the potency will be stated for only that form. Superoxide dismutase has been discussed elsewhere; it is available alone, combined with Vitamin E (though usually in the alpha form alone) and combined with other enzymes.

When these nutritional factors are used late in life, in the search for rejuvenation, rather than preventively, it is often helpful to add the enzymes which may improve digestive function. These include bromelain, pancreatic enzymes, and papaya. Bromelain, it should be noted, has two helpful actions: not only the help it gives in digesting protein, but an effect, like that of evening primrose oil, in stimulating the production of prostaglandin El.

ARTHRITIS

Don't skip this section because you're healthy. Sixty percent of my readers, according to life insurance actuaries, should live to be sixty-five or older. Sixty percent of those—one in every three of you now reading this book—will at that age have arthritis, hypertension, heart or kidney disease, hardening of the arteries, or some other unwelcome companion as they progress into what are called the "golden years." The diseases don't come out of the blue, and though they are concomitant with aging, they are not caused by time alone, for children have them, too, and some very old people don't. If aging were *the* cause, it would mean that your arthritic knee was somehow older than your healthy one. If stress, frequently blamed for osteoarthritis, were *the* cause, you would have to ask why there was more wear and tear in one shoulder than the other. All this means that the processes that cause such degenerative diseases begin long before the symptoms appear.

During many years of treating arthritis with niacinamide and other B complex vitamins, Dr. William Kaufman had the opportunity to watch the results when young, healthy people, free of arthritis, used the same vitamins. Though he significantly helped thousands of arthritics with vitamin therapy, he counted as his greatest achievement the discovery that arthritis could be barred and joints kept normal in those who applied his findings *preventively.*

There have been many claims made for diet in arthritis, most of which I shall not deal with. Some are sheer nonsense; some have limited usefulness; some would meet the needs of only a handful of arthritics; and none of these diets—including the one I am about to recommend—has universal application, which is to say that a panacea for arthritis doesn't exist. Those who have helped themselves by becoming vegetarians invariably will try to persuade all arthritics that this is *the* cure, forgetting that vegetarian animals and human beings do develop arthritis. Claims for copper bracelets are made by some arthritics who sincerely believe that wearing them has helped, but arthritis specialists find that at least some arthritics improve when their excessive blood copper levels are lowered. Claims made for green-tipped mussel extract are not adequately documented. However, there is a diet that has helped numerous arthritics. It involves not eating anything in the nightshade family. Thousands of case histories document its helpfulness, yet the Arthritis Foundation dismisses these as "anecdotal," the usual fate of any evidence gathered from case histories in the absence of double-blind controls.

That there are toxic constituents of foods is not a new and unproved idea. Parsnips, for instance, and perhaps such related vegetables as celery and parsley, contain significant amounts of chemicals that become toxic when exposed to light and that are mutagenic. This means that they are capable of altering heredity, invoking a possibility that they are cancer-producing. An ordinary portion of parsnip root could expose an individual to an amount of toxic chemicals that could cause some physiological effects under certain circumstances. Moreover, the idiosyncrasies of reactions to common foods, ranging from mild intolerance to severe allergy, have been reported in studies of arthritics whose symptoms worsened when they ate offending foods, or when they were exposed to chemicals or drugs to which they proved sensitive. For what reasons would the nightshades—a family of foods and weeds from which a number of poisons have been extracted—be exempt from suspicion? Cattle breeders have long known that weeds of the nightshade family can cause severe joint pains in cattle grazing upon them. (By the way, the cattle won't graze on nightshade unless they're starving.)

The no-nightshade diet involves eliminating four foods of that family: peppers (all types except black), potato, eggplant, and tomato. Tobacco, though obviously not an article of the diet, is also a nightshade, and should be eliminated. It sounds simple and easy to accomplish, but nightshades are ingredients of many processed foods, so the arthritic must read labels carefully, for some of the failures with the diet originate with continued and unsuspected consumption of these foods. Cheap yogurt, for instance, may be stiffened with potato starch, and paprika, a frequent offender for sensitive arthritics, may be listed on labels as "spice." Nonetheless, severely crippled arthritics have been freed from pain and their joint mobility improved by this diet. Less severe cases have enjoyed complete remission. The success rate in a number of types of arthritis, including the most common (osteoarthritis and rheumatoid arthritis), has been some 70 percent. Osteoarthritis, by far the most common, is a disorder that causes degeneration of bone and calcium deposits at the joints. Rheumatoid arthritis is caused by an abnormal functioning of the immune system, so that it attacks normal tissue. Some of the failures have been traced to unknowing continued consumption of nightshade foods. Some are induced by the continued use of medication that itself is a nightshade derivative, the anti-inflammatory agent Motrin being a classic example. The rest must represent individuals whose arthritis neither originates in nor is aggravated by nightshade chemicals.

Most unproved or "quack" remedies for arthritis are described by the medical orthodoxy as moneymaking rackets. Reading such sweeping generalizations, the public never pauses to ask who might profit financially by a ban on the consumption of potato, tomato, eggplant, and peppers. Moreover, those who discourage arthritics from trying the diet invariably utter not a word about the dangers of the drugs commonly prescribed. Unfortunately, the public never realizes that nightshade foods have been suspect for many centuries. The eggplant was known in the twelfth century as the "apple of insanity." The tomato was once called the "love apple," but before that, it was known as the "cancer apple." The potato was regarded with such suspicion that it became the target for the Society to Prevent Unnutritious Diet, from whose initials originated the word *spud*. And peppers and other spices have long been prohibited in diets for a number of human diseases.

A survey of American habits of nightshade consumption quickly reveals that we went on a dietary binge with these foods in the past quarter of a century. Years ago, tomato juice wasn't available, and Italian foods were an occasional treat. Previously, we peeled and boiled potatoes, thereby extracting much of the toxic chemical (solinase) in this food, which is concentrated near the skin (though present in the entire food). Now we bake potatoes and consume them with the skin. To give you a perspective on the toxicity of solinase, which is the mischief maker for some arthritics, consider extracting it from a year's intake of potato by an average American and giving it in one dose to a horse. The horse, an expert told me, would die.

Having watched many arthritics escape from the "prison of the disease," as one ex-sufferer put it, I know what questions will occur to my reader. Let me anticipate them.

1. What about the drugs I've been taking? Do I stop them when I go on the diet?

The best advice is to consult with the physician who prescribed the medications. They must be stopped because they interfere with the dividends from the diet, but it should be a slow withdrawal. However, if the drugs include nightshade factors of the belladonna and atropine type, the pace of withdrawal should be quick.

2. How long must I stay away from nightshades to test the results properly?

The duration of the arthritis and the age of the person are factors. Older people and more severe arthritics will take longer to respond. This isn't a hard and fast rule; we sometimes encounter surprises in a response in only a few days, but some people require months.

3. Are there any harmful effects from omitting these foods from the diet?

There is no indispensable food, and substitutions can be made for every nightshade. Sweet potato, which is really not a potato, can substitute for white potato. Any nutritious vegetable or fruit will take the place of tomato. Eggplant just isn't that important nutritionally. Peppers offer nothing nutritional that can't be had elsewhere in the diet, and their principal contributions are carotene (vegetable vitamin A) and vitamin C, both readily supplied by citrus and other fruits and vegetables.

4. A friend who tried the diet and benefited by it is puzzled by the quick and severe reaction he now gets with just a small amount of nightshade foods. When he was consuming large quantities of them and had arthritis, why wasn't he absolutely crippled?

The reaction to going back to nightshades perfectly parallels the experience of people who have been consuming large amounts of a food to which they then discover they are allergic. They avoid the food for a few months, and the symptoms, whatever they were, disappear. Then they discover that a very small portion of the offending food, far less than they previously ate, will start serious symptoms that they never noticed before. Apparently, when intake of a sensitizing food is large and regular, the body builds what immunity it can. When the food is withdrawn, the immune mechanism is retired from the scene, but when even a small amount of the offending food is then reintroduced, symptoms start. In the case of the nightshades, it often happens that an arthritic benefits from avoiding the large amounts previously consumed, and then reports that eating a dish containing even a minute amount of paprika, for example, will cause a flare-up of pain, stiffness, swelling, and impaired mobility of the joints. That experience has convinced many of the skeptical.

5. Does sensitivity to the nightshade foods play a part in any other disorders?

We suspect that it may be involved in myasthenia gravis and in diverticulosis and diverticulitis. The chemistry involved suggests that these foods may play a role in initiating or aggravating heart disease, but that is theoretical.

As one arthritic—who subsequently benefited significantly by avoiding these foods—remarked: "What did I have to lose in not eating white potato, eggplant, tomato, and peppers? Nothing but pain."

After writing what you have just read, I received an urgent note from Dr. Norman F. Childers, the research pioneer in the relationship of nightshade-food-sensitivity to arthritis. He reemphasized a point in his book on the subject, where a contributing expert noted that the nightshade foods contain vitamin D_3, which in animals may cause inflammation of the joints. Dr. Childers reported that responses to the no-nightshade diet are sometimes improved when the individual ceases to use milk products (which are universally fortified with vitamin D_3). He also observed that avoiding the vitamin brought responses in arthritics who had not responded at all to deletion of the nightshades from the diet. Fascinatingly, this, one of the several forms of the vitamin, is the type manufactured in the body by the action of sunshine on the skin, making it normal to our metabolism. It is possible, however, that the arthritics sensitive to it are not metabolizing it normally. The vitamin is normally converted to an active (hormone) form in the kidneys, a mechanism which, going awry, could permit abnormal accumulation of D_3 in the body. I called to Dr. Childers' attention the fact that in any group of patients given substantial doses of vitamin D_3, there will be a subgroup of abnormal reactors—i.e., individuals whose response includes an abnormal elevation of blood calcium, which, of course, could result in deposition of calcium at the joints. While the observation needs further research, it does suggest that avoiding vitamin D_3-enriched products might be rewarding for those who do not respond, or respond only partially to the avoidance of the nightshade foods.

Osteoarthritis

Dr. William Kaufman, the physician who developed the diet-vitamin therapy for osteoarthritis, practiced in Bridgeport, Connecticut, for many years. The benefits he brought to his patients are perhaps best, if indirectly, recognized by the fact that a letter addressed to "The Arthritis Doctor, Bridgeport" promptly reached him. Despite his success in rescuing arthritics who seemed hopelessly crippled, he carefully describes the limitations on his therapy. The treatment can cause significant improvement if the following conditions are met.

1. The patient must be eating a diet adequate in protein and calories.
2. The patient's joints must not have been excessively and thereby irreversibly damaged by his or her work or life-style.
3. The joints likewise must not have been so damaged by longstanding arthritis prior to treatment as to foreclose a chance for improvement.

To counter the skepticism of the orthodox rheumatologist, the background for this therapy should briefly be described. Many physicians will recall the pioneering research in nutrition of Dr. Tom Spies, who was honored by the American Medical Association (A.M.A.) for his contributions to the treatment of pellagra and other deficiency diseases. Two of his observations have disappeared from medical memory. He observed that patients with pellagra had joint pains that yielded to nutritional treatment. He also observed that for the lesser pains of arthritis, he could use vitamin therapy rather than the usual drugs. From these insights, Dr. William Kaufman took his inspiration for nutritional treatment of osteoarthritis. He demonstrated that osteoarthritis could not be successfully treated by correction of diet alone. Vitamin therapy in high doses was also necessary. This is not iconoclastic, for every competent nutritionist knows that recovery from persistent malnutrition requires greater intake of nutrients than is necessary for maintenance of the healthy body.

Dr. Kaufman's second contribution was prevention of degenerative disease at the joints.

Since there are those who insist that everyone, sick or well, can obtain needed vitamin intake from food alone, it is instructive to observe eleven of Dr. Kaufman's arthritic patients who were of that persuasion and refused to take vitamin therapy. They insisted that the doctor place them on the "best possible diet." He complied, but none of them enjoyed an improvement in the use of their joints. There were others who reduced their prescribed doses of niacinamide or who substituted an ordinary multiple vitamin supplement of the "one-a-day" variety; and whatever benefits they had achieved from the niacinamide treatment faded away. Those patients who refused to continue the niacinamide therapy, after participating in it for a significant length of time, likewise suffered a gradual worsening of their joint disabilities until they returned to the degree of impairment they had before receiving niacinamide treatment.

Because the basic concept behind the Recommended Dietary Allowances troubles me—I am, in fact, appalled by generalizations about human nutritional requirements, particularly when the human level is much lower than the amount stipulated for monkeys and pigs—I don't propose to quote the RDA for niacinamide. You can find that elsewhere, if you must. It is a fraction of the amount that a paper published in the *Journal of the American Medical Association* described as "improving the condition of a normal mouth"—an utterance that has long intrigued me, since it implies not only that we cannot accurately define a normal mouth, but that achieving it requires much more niacinamide than the A.M.A. Council on Foods has ever admitted we need. The range of requirements for protein acids (amino acids) for human beings is up to fivefold the low RDA figure. That range holds for calcium, likewise, and for many other nutrients. It would seem to be a good investment for young adults to keep their niacinamide intake at the 50-mg. mark, which is about four times the "authoritative" figure.

The doses used in niacinamide therapy for arthritis are quite high, and Dr. Kaufman urges that self-medication should not be attempted. His therapy starts with 1,500 mg. daily, in six doses, for slight joint dysfunction, and increases for moderate, severe, and extremely severe joint involvement, up to a high of 4,000 mg. daily. It is emphasized that doses must be divided, not taken all at once, for maintenance of the blood level of the vitamin is critical if results are to be obtained. In some cases, Dr. Kaufman has found added dividends from prescribing other factors of the vitamin B complex, to accompany the niacinamide. He makes correction of the diet mandatory. I should be inclinded to make supplementing with vitamin B_6 mandatory when high doses of niacinamide are used, for there is a relationship between the two factors, and, as you will read a little later, some physicians have found vitamin B_6 and potassium helpful in osteoarthritis.

The golfer with severe arthritis of the wrists and the aged woman who more or less pulls herself upstairs by grasping the banister will find that their habits nullify the benefits of the Kaufman therapy. Just as one gives a broken leg time to mend, so must arthritics allow time for their joints to heal.

I should like to add that as a seasoned observer of the medical and nutritional scene, I found Dr. Kaufman's research so important (and so much neglected) that I proposed him for the honor of the Tom Spies Memorial Lecture at the International Academy of Preventive Medicine. This by way of preface to an admonition: If your arthritis is troublesome and progressing, find a physician who will be open-minded (if not curious) enough to supervise this vitamin therapy for you. Medical nutritionists are likely to cooperate, and, if you do not have a physician at present, you can write to one of the societies listed in the Appendix to obtain referral to such a practitioner.

Vis-à-vis the role of niacinamide in preventing arthritis, you may be interested in a simple home test that may, though you're now healthy (or think you are), tell you that the process which one day will emerge as osteoarthritis is already at work. It is a test of balance and *must not be conducted without someone observing you as you try it,* for it involves a possible fall. In a standing position, close your eyes and raise your knee, clasping it with your hands, until your thigh is parallel to the floor. If you fall, this may mean that a deficiency of niacinamide, while not yet contributing to osteoarthritis, has already affected your sense of balance.

Throughout this discussion of the Kaufman treatment, I have written nothing concerning types of arthritis other than osteoarthritis. In one of his papers, and in conversations with me, the physician made it clear that rheumatoid arthritis is much more complicated than the other types, because of the witch's brew of allergy, glandular, and immunological disturbances that plays a role in it, but niacinamide is nonetheless often helpful to these patients as well, for the good reason that rheumatoid arthritis very frequently involves some degree of osteoarthritis, too.

Rheumatoid Arthritis

The acronym I keep in mind when discussing rheumatoid arthritis is SAID. It stands for Stress, Allergy, Immunology, and Deficiency. The story of the standard approach to this disease is the usual one of drug therapy and neglect of the dietary factors that contribute to rheumatoid arthritis.

This neglect is more than unforgivable; it is astonishing, because the history of rheumatic disorders was linked to nutrition almost seventy-five years ago. It was observed during World War I that the "bully beef" eaten by British troops conferred resistance to trench fever, while American troops, whose snacks were doughnuts and coffee, were much more susceptible to the disease. American children with rheumatic fever much later were also found to have a high sugar intake and low protein in their diet. Particularly striking was the absence of eggs in their diet, an observation that led to a trial of eggs versus penicillin therapy for the disease. Given two eggs daily, the children improved more than the control group, whose treatment was the classical one—penicillin. That lesson, though, slipped from the memory of medicine and, in any case, was not applied to the problems of the rheumatoid arthritic. Though I have already expressed my wariness of the sweeping generalizations in diet, I must record my observation that many of the patients with rheumatoid arthritis do best on a diet moderately low in carbohydrates (starch and sugar), adequate in protein, and rich in polyunsaturated fat—sunflower seed oil particularly. It has been overlooked that this oil is immunosuppressive, which is to say that it may be helpful in restraining the immune system when it is overzealous and attacks normal tissues and cells, a situation that occurs in rheumatoid arthritis.

Many of these patients profit by large doses of vitamin C. "Large" in this context means a dosage determined by the physician, which falls just short of causing loose bowel movements and diarrhea. The doctor arrives at this by gradually raising the intake of the vitamin until the laxative effect is demonstrated, then reducing the dose just below this point. This point, termed "titration to diarrhea," differs widely among patients. The diarrhea that results from going beyond the patient's tolerance for vitamin C is often given as an example of the toxicity of the vitamin. It is difficult to believe that so ignorant a comment would be repeated by competent physicians.

Pantothenic acid may be helpful because it stimulates the adrenal gland, a property of importance in the treatment of a disease in which poor adrenal function has been noted. In fact, Kendall, the discoverer of cortisone, once remarked that uneven tides of production of the hormone might contribute to rheumatoid arthritis. Acting on this thesis, British physicians experimented with the administration of pantothenic acid. They elicited favorable reactions, but found that increasing doses did not raise the blood levels beyond a certain limit. In the effort to pass through that ceiling, they gave the arthritics doses of "royal jelly," the food created by bees for their queen. The theory was that there is so much pantothenic acid in royal jelly that possibly other factors were present which might improve utilization. The theory was right: With the royal jelly, the invisible "ceiling" on blood levels of pantothenic acid yielded. As blood concentrations of the vitamin increased, so did the benefits, though, of course, there was a point of diminishing returns. That research is gathering dust in the medical libraries, and in the past quarter of a century, I have never met a patient of an orthodox rheumatologist who had been given the chance to try the pantothenic acid and royal jelly therapy, though it is free of side reactions. At any rate, while it may be difficult to locate sources of royal jelly, some apiaries do sell it, and at least one company has marketed it for some years. It is important that royal jelly be unprocessed, meaning that it must not be dried (desiccated).

Zinc has proved to be a critical nutrient for many rheumatoid arthritics. Zinc deficiency is frequent in this disorder, and the administration of zinc supplements has proved markedly beneficial.

The rheumatoid arthritic, it follows, may benefit markedly by a reduction of processed carbohydrates in the diet and by attention to the intake of eggs, zinc, vitamin C, pantothenic acid, and, as you will discover later in this section, octocosanol, selenium, superoxide dismutase, and vitamin B_{12}. Very important in this disorder is testing for allergies. What follows is a discussion of allergy in the narrow context of arthritis. In the section on allergy you will find expanded information on other aspects of allergy, including some testing methods recently introduced.

Allergy in Arthritis

Just as the arthritis establishment fails to recognize the effectiveness of nutritional therapies in these diseases, so has it been blind to the role that food and drug and chemical allergies may play in rheumatoid arthritis. Yet a study confirming that role was published more than thirty years ago. In it, the physicians reported that patients improved when allergenic foods were removed from their diets. In part, orthodox allergists contributed to this cultural lag, for, astonishingly, while they are convinced that allergy to pollen, dust, and molds is real, many suspect food allergies are "iffy" or too difficult to prove. Yet a recent study conceded that eating sensitizing foods or being exposed to certain chemicals can significantly worsen rheumatoid arthritis. The corollary was also demonstrated: Avoiding the offending substances was shown to produce a "state of complete disease remission" in some patients.

The average patient reacted to some seven foods of about thirty-one that were tested. The most frequent troublemakers were cereals and grains; red meats came second. Generally, few patients had reactions to vegetables and fruits, but the reactions of individual patients were exactly that—individual.

Of twenty-four patients fed foods containing additives and contaminants, thirteen reacted with symptoms, four of these so badly affected that they couldn't complete the planned schedule of six such meals. Of nineteen patients who inhaled the by-products of burning natural gas, fourteen suffered aggravation of arthritis symptoms. Seven in seventeen had an adverse reaction to formaldehyde, and all but one of these developed arthritic symptoms. Six of fifteen reacted to the vapor of chlorine, three of these developing symptoms of arthritis, and five of fifteen developed arthritic symptoms when insecticide was tested. In several of the patients, all symptoms of arthritis disappeared as long as they stayed away from the sensitizing food or chemical.

There is pertinency in bringing you this information. The odds are 100 to 1 that the average rheumatoid arthritic has never been tested for allergy as part of his or her troubles. The estimate is safe, for when I have queried audiences consisting of 500 arthritics, only one hand has been raised in response to the question "How many of you ever have been tested for allergy to foods, additives, chemicals, and drugs?"

There is a small group of allergists who explore the entire external and internal environments for sources of allergic reactions, not only in arthritics, of course. They are known as bioecological allergists, and you will find their society listed in the Appendix as a source of referral if you find that necessary. These practitioners often use vitamins B_6 and C in high doses to help calm allergic reactions, often with a rotation diet that is arranged so that you do not repeat favorite foods often enough to initiate or perpetuate allergic reactions. They are distinguished, too, by their use of testing methods more satisfactory and reliable that the ancient "scratch" tests, which give too many false positives and false negatives. These include the cytotoxic, RAST (radioallergosorbent test), Rinkel, and sublingual challenge methods. If you are a rheumatoid arthritic, bioecological allergists may have a great deal to offer you. If you have another type of arthritis, it is less likely but still possible that allergic reactions are increasing your troubles. To anticipate a question, the sensitivity to nightshades, in the light of what you have read, can be an allergic reaction in some individuals, but appears to be a toxic one in others.

Nutrients Important to the Arthritic

Pantothenic Acid □   Pantothenic acid, which may be listed on vitamin labels as "pantothenol" or calcium pantothenate, was originally isolated and synthesized by one of my professional friends, Dr. Roger Williams. He has long been convinced that estimates of requirements for pantothenic acid have been far too low, and often has suggested that 50 mg. daily would be a realistic goal in preventive nutrition. Doses used in the British research described earlier were far higher, and your physician should set the therapeutic amount. He will find, in the medical literature, research by Esther Tuttle, M.D., clearly indicating that pantothenic acid supplementation increases resistance to stress, an action important to rheumatoid arthritics.

Selenium □   For many years, selenium was mistakenly regarded as a nuisance, a threat to health, a poison, and a possible cause of cancer. It took years of research to demonstrate that selenium is both normal and vital to the body, and that it helps to create an enzyme that, like superoxide dismutase (SOD), is an important defense against activated oxygen of the type which can accelerate aging and contribute to cancer. As usual, veterinarians capitalized upon selenium's usefulness long before it was administered to human beings. Since selenium interlocks with vitamin E in antioxidant effects, veterinarians have long used a formula that contains 1,000 mcg. (1 mg.) of selenium, accompanied by 68 I.U. (International Units) of vitamin E, which markedly relieved arthritic pain and swelling in animals. Finally applied to human arthritis, selenium therapy "moderated the progression of the disease." It has been reported to be useful in several types of human arthritis, including rheumatoid arthritis, osteoarthritis, and the type caused by physical injury to a joint. In the treatment of the last, vitamins A, C, and E were used with the selenium and proved to relieve pain in the injured joints. This is not merely a painkilling action, like that of aspirin; it is a contribution to healing.

There is still a hangover from the ancient but mistaken belief that selenium in any quantity is dangerous. Actually, the Japanese woman's relative immunity to breast cancer, which she loses when she moves to America, has been traced to the higher intake of selenium provided by the emphasis on fish in the traditional Japanese diet. The Japanese intake hovers around 500 mcg. (0.5 mg.) daily; ours is more likely to be somewhere between 200 and 300 mcg. daily, a deficit we owe to overprocessing of food and infrequent use of seafood. A supplement of selenium that would make sense, therefore, would be somewhere between 50 mcg. and 100 mcg. daily. This should not be in the form of sodium selenite, but as organically bound selenium, such as the form in which it occurs in yeast. Yeast tablets specifically enriched in organically bound selenium are available. The therapeutic range of dosage goes from 200 mcg. to 500 mcg. daily, and in the actual treatment of terminal cancer, as much as 2 mg. (2,000 mcg.) daily has been the dose. Cases of terminal lung cancer benefited, and autopsies on those who died revealed no toxic effect of selenium. This, however, does not license the reader for self-treatment with this mineral, for the risk of an overdose is real.

Superoxide Dismutase (SOD) ☐ Superoxide dismutase, in a copper-and-zinc form, is natural to the body and is a powerful member of a group of biological antioxidants. Although oxygen is a necessity for life, under certain circumstances it becomes hyperactive, in which form it attacks the structure and function of cells, impairs their chemistry, and thereby may speed aging, contribute to disease, and even cause cancer. Ironically, superoxide dismutase is better known to veterinarians than to physicians. It is now being tested, with early results that are promising, in human rheumatoid arthritis and osteoarthritis, but verterinarians have long used it to treat enlarged prostate in dogs and arthritis in large animals such as horses. Among the latter was Seattle Slew, whose brilliant racing career was jeopardized by a threatening, progressive arthritis. This magnificent animal was treated with SOD, which conquered the disease, and he returned to racing to win the triple crown. Through the years when veterinarians were thoroughly acquainted with the usefulness of SOD in arthritis therapy, it was ignored by those who treat the human form of the disease. It is an ancient observation of nutritionists that animals receive better nutritional care and therapy than human beings. It isn't that we need less; obviously, it is that the animals have a cash value.

Superoxide dismutase is sold in health food stores, for dose by mouth. In this form, it may have some usefulness as a protection against activated oxygen and the mischief it causes. However, the blood levels reachable by oral dosage aren't high enough to be really useful in treating arthritis. Injections are far more efficient, and the medical nutritionist may combine the two methods, using the doses by mouth to help to maintain the blood levels of the enzyme achieved by injection. Label directions for the use of superoxide dismutase are supplementary amounts. The medical nutritionist may wish to recommend higher doses for therapy. In rheumatoid arthritis, it has been found to be as effective as gold therapy, without its dangers.

Vitamin B_{12} ☐   Though vitamin B_{12} is inextricably identified with its role in avoiding pernicious anemia and the disturbances of the nervous system and brain deficiency that it can cause, the vitamin has other properties that are useful in arthritis. In bursitis, coupled with physiotherapy such as ultrasonic, vitamin B_{12} helps in relieving pain. In arthritis of every type, fatigability is one of the inevitable associated symptoms. It seems little known that this vitamin has an effective energizing action, which has been demonstrated in definitive research.

Absorption of vitamin B_{12} taken by mouth is poor, and for that reason it is usually given by injection. There are two alternatives or supplements to injections for administration of vitamin B_{12}. Desiccated stomach tissue, which contains a factor promoting the utilization of the vitamin, is sometimes given with oral doses of it. Another and more effective method is the use of lozenges containing the vitamin in 500 mcg. or 1,000 mcg. designed to be dissolved under the tongue. The blood vessel network there is profuse, and absorption is fast. The reader will recall that nitroglycerin, used as a heart medicine, is effectively administered by that route.

The supplementary dose of vitamin B_{12}, in sublingual lozenges, is 500 mcg. to 1,000 mcg. daily. The medical nutritionist may substantially increase that for therapeutic purposes, to as much as 5 mg. daily, using lesser amounts if the oral administration is a sustaining dose between injections of the vitamin. If the dietary history, with particular reference to green vegetables, milk, and liver, is poor, a supplementary intake of folic acid, used simultaneously with the vitamin B_{12}, is advisable.

Vitamin C ☐   Although highly dangerous drugs are prescribed for arthritics without criticism from the medical establishment, every effort has been made to discourage the use of large doses of vitamin C. I should consider discussing these as a waste of time, were it not for the very real risk that you and your physician, exposed to this propaganda, may concur in depriving you of the possible benefits of high intake of the vitamin, not only in arthritis, but in other disorders.

Dr. Victor Herbert reported that high blood levels of vitamin C destroy vitamin B_{12}, thereby creating a risk of pernicious anemia. Unfortunately, the competent researchers who found Dr. Herbert's research to be based on faulty laboratory tests do not seem to gain access to the newspapers as this professional antivitamin propagandist does. There are at least three papers contradicting Herbert's statement, all of them published in journals of excellent scientific reputation.

Other reports, linking vitamin C with oxalate kidney stone formation, have likewise been refuted, and the vitamin in large doses has been found to be safe for those with normal kidney function. Sterility in women has been attributed to a high intake of the vitamin, though orthomolecular psychiatrists who have prescribed megadoses for schizophrenic women—as much as 60 gm. daily, and for very long periods—have seen no interference with reproduction.

The effectiveness of vitamin C in preventing or mitigating colds and allergies has likewise been challenged, though my own observations over a period of nearly forty years indicate that for some people, the vitamin is quite effective. This subject is dealt with elsewhere in this text.

I have mentioned one "adverse" report on vitamin C that happens to be accurate and yet misleading. This is the action of high doses in causing diarrhea. The report is accurate, but the reaction is actually used to gauge the individual's tolerance for the highest possible dose. In the medical nutritionist's technique, moderate doses of vitamin C by mouth are gradually increased to the point where the patient reports softening of the stool or outright diarrhea. The dose is then lowered to the one just short of that which caused the laxative effect.

There are many ways in which generous supplies of vitamin C, which must be used in the form of ascorbic acid (not sodium ascorbate, which would be taboo for those on a low-salt diet), can be helpful to the arthritic. The actions of vitamin C include its beneficial effect on the immune system, which malfunctions in rheumatoid arthritis, as it does in numerous other disorders. The vitamin is involved in the synthesis of collagen, which might be described as the glue that binds our cells together; and in arthritis, disturbances of collagen are frequent. In septic arthritis, where there is an underlying infection, vitamin C serves to help the white blood cells in attacking the invader. In viral infections, such as serum hepatitis, it has proved to be a superb treatment, eliminating the dangers of blood transfusions as a vehicle for infection. Hepatitis patients treated with vitamin C recover more quickly. Ankylosing spondylitis, a crippling form of arthritis, was reported to be checked by large doses of vitamin C in a book written by a patient, Norman Cousins, who attributed the success of his therapy to a zest for life and a good sense of humor.

Dr. Linus Pauling, whose intractable tendency toward frequent, severe colds was overcome with the vitamin, has set a range, rather than a figure, for optimal intake of vitamin C: from 250 mg. to 2,500 mg. daily. The latter is the amount we humans would synthesize if our bodies could manufacture the vitamin as most animals can. The therapeutic dose can be enormous in hepatitis and schizophrenia and other grave diseases. In certain instances, it is preferable that it be administered intravenously, but in any case, a medical nutritionist should supervise when vitamin C in very high doses is being used for therapy. In some instances, these may be as high as 100 g. daily or more.

Octocosanol ☐ Octocosanol is a long-chain, waxy alcohol, found naturally in wheat germ oil, and originally used to promote muscle tone and resistance to muscular fatigue both in athletes and in subjects who were in poor physical condition. It is described elsewhere in this text as part of the treatments for brain injury and for nerve-muscle disorders such as multiple sclerosis. Only recently, I received reports that arthritics had benefited by octocosanol therapy, which makes sense in the light of their muscle pains, weakness, and spasms. Octocosanol is best used as a supplement in its natural vehicle: wheat germ oil. Label instructions usually lead to one capsule daily, yielding 2 milligrams of the factor. Therapeutic doses range from 1 mg. to 10 mg. or more daily. In these high dosages, the medical nutritionist often must cope with patients who tolerate octocosanol, as most do, but do not tolerate such large amounts of oil. In such cases, he is likely to recommend tablets of crystalline octocosanol, which are available in high potencies, and accompany them with wheat germ oil or, in very malnourished, elderly, or alcoholic patients, with evening primrose oil. The latter oil is not used arbitrarily, for it is both scarce and costly, but does offer advantages for patients who have difficulty in utilizing the type of fatty acid found in other oils.

Evening Primrose Oil ☐ There is a hormone, produced as needed in the body, which has anti-inflammation actions, and stimulates circulation—effects obviously important to arthritics. The production of this hormone is dependent upon a nutritional factor which is extremely rare in ordinary foods, but is provided in generous amounts by evening primrose oil. The oil, however, will not contribute to the synthesis of the hormone if the diet is not adequate, if there is an excessive intake of alcohol or the trans fats found in partially hydrogenated oils (used in many food products), or if there is an inadequate amount of insulin. These chemistries are discussed fully on page 154.

The nutritional effort may be rewarding. It has been for some arthritics, but it has been said there is more primrose oil being sold than is produced, which means that failures with the therapy may derive from unknowing use of a substitute oil which is necessarily ineffective. You must patronize a reliable supplier.

Olive Oil ☐ Some rheumatoid arthritics have benefited from increased intake of olive oil. This is largely inexplicable, since olive oil does not have the same characteristics as the polyunsaturated oils with which the medical profession has been preoccupied. It may be due to suppression of the immune system, which in rheumatoid arthritis is misbehaving.

THE AUTISTIC CHILD

The autistic child's troubles may originate with an excess of ammonia in the brain. That, a metabolic problem, can be treated. He may have nutritional deficiencies; indeed, if they occur frequently in normal children, why would the autistic child be exempt? He may have hypoglycemia. He may be reacting adversely to common foods that are innocuous for the rest of the family.

Confronting and solving these problems may not give you a normal child, but freeing him of them *must* yield significant improvement. You need a sympathetic pediatrician who is also a bioecological allergist, competent in nutrition and neurology, and the management of hypoglycemia. The Appendix guides you to sources of referral for some of these specialities, though I must warn you that pediatric nutritionists are far scarcer than pediatricians ready to prescribe tranquilizers. It should make the journey more tolerable if I tell you that I have seen doses of one single vitamin—B$_6$—radically normalize some of these children. The problems are usually more complex, but the dividends make the effort to identify and solve them worthwhile.

In the Introduction, I voiced my distaste for the insistence on double-blind tests for sick people. Applied to children, they are doubly infuriating. Applied to autistic children? The answer should be obvious. Yet consider this history, which I received from Dr. William Philpott, an orthomolecular psychiatrist: The patients were identical twins, both autistic. Diagnosed at Albert Einstein Medical School, the twins were often displayed at neurological conferences, as interesting examples of what obviously must be a genetic factor in autism. The mother encountered Dr. Philpott, who examined the twins for nutritional deficiencies, of which he found seven, identical in kind but not in degree; and for cerebral allergy, again identical in kind but not in degree. He corrected the children's nutrition. Months later, Albert Einstein Medical School again requested that the mother bring the twins to a neurological symposium. She consented, but told the neurologist that the twins were playing with each other and with other children; that they were talking, responding to affection, and going to school as educable youngsters. The neurologist wanted to know how that was accomplished, and when the mother told him about Dr. Philpott's investigation and treatment, his comment threw a blinding light on the dark areas of the dogma-locked mind. "You can't do that," he protested. "It has to be double blind!" One would have to be doubly blind, as the parent or the physician of an autistic child, to deny possible help from harmless therapy on the basis of such unreasoning medical prejudice.

Some autistic children, by the action of a metabolic error, have abnormal levels of ammonia in their brains. Such a metabolic error can be managed, if not banished. Some of them—perhaps a large percentage—have a faulty link in their enzyme chemistries, to which therapy can be applied with vitamin B_6. Some of them need both the vitamin and supplements of a sulfur-containing amino acid. All of them deserve the chance to escape from the bizarre world in which they live.

In the Appendix, you will find the name and address of a San Diego psychologist who has done more for autistic children than anyone in his field: not with reward-and-punishment behavioral conditioning, but with nutrients. Your physician can obtain valuable information from Dr. Bernard Rimland's small institute. I urge you to give your autistic child the benefit of the exchange of that information.

BRAIN DAMAGE

See the discussion of cerebral palsy, page 30, and the Epilogue. The therapies described in these sections apply to traumatic brain damage (physical injury), post-stroke symptoms, carbon monoxide poisoning, and other chemical insults to the brain.

BURNING MOUTH AND TONGUE

Constant burning of the mouth is sometimes traced to deficiency in vitamin B_{12}. Treatment with oral doses of the vitamin is often unsuccessful, because absorption of the vitamin by that route is poor. This is sometimes overcome by giving dried stomach tissue with the vitamin B_{12}, since it contains a factor that promotes absorption of the vitamin. The physician may sidestep these problems, and usually does, by administering the vitamin by injection. The medical nutritionist may also use injections, but may substitute for them, or augment their effect by prescribing, lozenges of vitamin B_{12} to be dissolved under the tongue. I find that many failures with this therapy are based on inadequate dosage, whether orally administered or by injection. Label instructions are often inadequate. Needless to say, a tongue or mouth that is burning because of a lack of vitamin B_{12} invites investigation to determine if lack of hydrochloric acid in the stomach or pernicious anemia are behind the deficiency.

Other causes of hot tongue and mouth are deficiency in niacinamide, a need for a higher intake of the entire vitamin B complex, an allergy to toothpaste or the ingredients in chewing gum, and a sensitivity or allergy to the plastics of dentures. Emotional factors, such as stress and depression, can also disturb the mouth in this way.

The average person worries about a coated tongue; the nutritionist worries about a bare and shiny one. Coating can come from mouth breathing, from food regurgitated in sleep, or from smoking, while the bare tongue, particularly when its color is magenta rather than the normal red, often is a token of deficiency in vitamin B complex. In addition to the usual B-complex concentrate, desiccated liver is a very useful supplement when the tongue is bare or cracked. (This does not apply to cracks that are present from birth.) The liver concentrate is also essential in some types of gingivitis (inflammation of the gums). Niacinamide therapy has been helpful for gingivitis, burning tongue, and hot mouth. This vitamin also helps to reduce tartar deposits on the teeth.

BURNS AND SUNBURN

Though I have seen no evidence that the hospital burn centers have yet discovered it, there is no remedy for burns more effective than the contents of a few capsules of mixed tocopherols (vitamin E). For burns not requiring medical attention, including sunburn, simply clip the end of the capsule, and squeeze the contents on the burned area. If you react as most people do, the quickness of the relief and healing will startle you. The application should be renewed every three or four hours.

Aloe Vera juice is a useful and soothing adjunct to the Vitamin E treatment.

CARPAL TUNNEL SYNDROME

*T*his is a disease of the hands, causing intense numbness, tingling, swelling, and, if chronic, muscular weakness or atrophy. In long-standing cases, there may be involvement of the shoulder, so that the disease is sometimes called "shoulder-hand syndrome." It has been blamed on pressure on a nerve. However, thanks to the research of Dr. John Ellis, we have learned that deficiency in vitamin B_6 (pyridoxine)—a deficiency very common in American diets—can cause this painful condition. Evidence for the role of the deficiency came from observing pregnant women, who often have swelling of the hands and feet and sometimes show clear evidence of carpal tunnel syndrome. Since in pregnancy there is a heightened requirement for the vitamin, which unfortunately may coincide with that stage of pregnancy when morning sickness interferes with food intake, it was not unexpected that vitamin B_6 would promptly relieve carpal tunnel syndrome in expectant mothers. Pertinent is the fact that the same vitamin has been used to treat one type of morning sickness in pregnancy.

In some individuals where the condition has existed for a long time, the painful shoulder involvement takes much longer to respond than does the condition of the hands. Six weeks of vitamin B_6 treatment often eliminates swelling and pain in the hands, but the painful shoulder may take months, and some residual discomfort may remain. The critical factor is the duration of the condition before the vitamin therapy is started. Long-term disability may have caused muscular atrophy, which is not reversed by this vitamin therapy. Birth control pills can cause a deficiency in B_6, and trigger the disorder.

Although many disorders require megadoses of vitamins for treatment, it is noteworthy that Dr. Ellis reported that he had achieved results with moderate intake of vitamin B_6—ranging between 50 mg. and 100 mg. daily. The medical nutritionist may wish to increase that by a considerable margin, using five to ten times as much. It may be necessary to continue the B_6 supplementing for a lifetime.

CEREBRAL PALSY

My experience with cerebral palsy is largely with the spastic type. I have no nutritional panacea for it, but there is an approach that may interest you. It utilizes octocosanol, vitamin E, and the vitamin B complex, high in inositol. The initial case was that of a six-year-old boy, a spastic, who was brought to the Massachusetts Bay State Training Center to be measured for a back brace to check a deformity developing as a result of the atrophy of the muscles. His mother persuaded the physician to consult with me. I informed him that I had no experience with cerebral palsy but that I had found octocosanol to be useful in a number of nerve-muscle disorders and, barring allergy, to be harmless. I suggested he try it. He agreed, asking me to give the mother the necessary information and instruct her to start the therapy as soon as possible. The boy returned to the institution a month later to be fitted with the brace. It did not fit, and examination showed a growth of muscle tissue which, since there had been no exercise (nor any possible), had to be a result of the octocosanol therapy. He instructed the mother to continue it. She was to send duplicate reports to the physician and to me. The seventh monthly report said: "Danny was helping me to dry dishes last night, and put one down too near the edge of the table. It fell, but he caught it before it hit the floor. He went down doing it, but what he was able to do tells you how much he has improved."

I made a number of attempts to interest the cerebral palsy societies in exploring the possibilities of this and accompanying nutritional therapies in the disorder. I encountered no interest, and sometimes active hostility. I am still prepared to send your physician the protocol on request. No drugs are involved, and no side effects other than a slight sedative effect on an occasional child or infrequent allergic reactions. The latter are usually predictable in that they occur only in highly allergic individuals. Though I write of children with cerebral palsy, I also include adults, though I believe the prognosis is better with younger patients. The physician can address me in care of the International Academy of Preventive Medicine at the address supplied in the Appendix (page 176).

COLD SORES, SHINGLES, AND GENITAL HERPES

It has well been said that the disorder for which there are many remedies has no cure. The description certainly applies to persistent "cold sores" and to shingles, but *not* to genital herpes, regardless of what you may have heard before.

Lysine, an amino acid, has been effective against cold sores for many sufferers. The action is predicated upon the antagonism between this amino acid and another, arginine, which the herpes virus needs. When the lysine intake is raised, the virus is frequently prevented from taking over cells and nudging them into producing more virus. So it is that canker sores, cold sores, and similar lesions of the gums and mouth have been successfully treated with lysine. It usually is available in 500-mg. tablets. The amount specified on the label may satisfy your physician, but medical nutritionists frequently will prescribe more.

Another nutrient that has both topical and systemic effects against both cold sores and shingles is vitamin B_{12}. Injections of the vitamin are frequently necessary, though there has been success in the use of sublingual lozenges of the vitamin, used either as the sole treatment or to sustain blood levels between injections. Both orthodox physicians and medical nutritionists, in my experience, tend to underdose the vitamin, particularly in the injection form. I find that some individuals do not respond until the injected dose reaches as high as 50 mg., which for this vitamin is very high. Such a dose, however, has been used, with other B vitamins, in the successful treatment of diabetic neuropathy, so there is a precedent for use of such a potent level.

Another observation, which is mine alone: If the injectable solution of vitamin B_{12}, usually 1 mg. per cubic centimeter, is applied topically to cold sores and shingles, it markedly stimulates healing and relieves itching and pain. Applications every four hours are effective in many cases. This is, of course, an adjunct treatment that can and should be combined with the lysine or other treatments.

"Other treatments" include an effective one that has been neglected by the professions, though papers reporting it have appeared in prestigious journals. This is the treatment with adenosine-

5-monophosphate (My-B-Den), which is a phosphorous compound natural to the body and important in energy metabolism. It is also useful in cold sores and shingles but, more remarkably, is effective against genital herpes, with one proviso: It must be used when the infection is active. Genital herpes tends to go into resting or "latent" inactive stages during which the treatment will not affect it. When lesions are present, the adenosine treatment should be used. It is available in sublingual lozenges but is more effective in the injectable form, with the lozenges used between injections to sustain the action. The use of vitamin B_{12} injections simultaneously enhances the therapeutic effect. If your physician is interested, he can obtain information from the man who pioneered in this research: Dr. S. H. Sklar.*

THE COMMON COLD

Everyone knows what causes colds: getting chilled or running into a virus or some unfriendly bacteria. Unfortunately, what everyone "knows" isn't true. If not the dominant source of colds, then a large factor is allergy. Often, we don't catch colds—we eat them, and the person who denies being allergic and simultaneously admits to many colds is simply making a good case for the need for tests for allergy.

You have probably heard that vitamin C neither prevents nor aborts colds. For some people, that's true. For others, vitamin C is a blessing. If it doesn't prevent all their colds, it is effective sometimes, and at least it shortens the duration, reduces the frequency, and lowers the level of symptoms. Why shouldn't it? Vitamin C is an antihistamine—and so are the drugs widely advertised for colds and for nasal congestion. However, the vitamin has another action, of importance in any infection: It aids the white blood cells in their normal function of fighting bacteria. I suspect, also, that it blocks the receptors used by viruses to gain entrance to cells, thereby not kill-

* See Appendix (p. 177) for address.

ing the virus, but preventing it from reproducing. Otherwise, it's difficult to explain the effectiveness of the vitamin in hepatitis and other viral infections.

Despite the public's facile explanations of what causes colds, there are types that don't fit. There is, for instance, an emotional cold, deriving from sexual frustration or from bottled-up anger that can't be expressed. (The nose—if you've forgotten the purpose of perfume—is a sex organ.)

When asked to specify the dose of vitamin C needed to abort a cold, a medical nutritionist made a logical but somewhat startling reply. "Is it," he asked, "a ten-gram cold? A fifty-gram cold? A hundred-gram cold?" In other words, dose is set by the severity of the condition.

Up to this point, you have probably read what medical nutritionists learned from the research of Dr. Linus Pauling and those who preceded him. What I am about to write derives from my own observations.

Years ago, Dr. C. Ward Crampton published a paper in the *N.Y. State Journal of Medicine,* reporting his experience in prescribing large doses of vitamin A for colds. The paper recorded a year of observation, involving many patients; yet the good doctor was so cautious that he compelled the journal to hold his manuscript for another year, before publication, to be sure that his later experience confirmed his earlier finding. It did; and yet the paper has been ignored ever since.

In the 1940s, Dr. Carl Zoll and I were experimenting with vitamin A in a type of tuberculosis. In that research, we observed an antagonism between this vitamin and ascorbic acid. Vitamin A was an effective treatment for the pneumonia associated with lung tuberculosis; vitamin C appeared to activate the infection. When I transferred these observations to the common cold, the same phenomenon appeared—in *some* people. There were those whose colds responded to vitamin C but were unaffected by vitamin A. There were those who responded to vitamin A but became distinctly worse when shifted to vitamin C. The tendency in the latter group was for the cold to drop from the head into the chest, producing a lingering bronchitis. And there were those who responded to neither vitamin, as there were colds which didn't, even in patients whose previous colds had.

I learned from this that it is very necessary to learn whether one is a vitamin C responder or a vitamin A responder (or, unhappily, neither). If you take vitamin A, and you're a vitamin C candidate, nothing happens. If you take vitamin C when you should be taking vitamin A, you may drop the cold down and wind up with bronchitis. Obviously, if you don't know which type you are, you start with vitamin A, the worst penalty then being failure.

An average (not devastating) cold may respond to 10 g. of vitamin C daily, taken until symptoms disappear. The vitamin A responder will take the vitamin for five days, in a dose of 250,000 units daily. (The period is too short for toxicity.) Warning: When your cold is suppressed, don't go into full activity, for fatigue will reawaken the symptoms.

It is important to use the vitamin at the first sign of the cold. This may not be a stuffed nose. It may be fatigue, or loss of normal buoyancy, or tightness or pain of the scalp. Know thyself.

CROHN'S DISEASE (REGIONAL ILEITIS)

Some years ago, at a medical symposium, I heard Dr. Wilfred Shute report on the treatment of regional ileitis with the highest dose of vitamin E I have ever heard discussed: 16,000 units daily. He said follow-up X-ray showed complete recovery with the patient symptom-free. One case does not a therapy make, but the history might keep us alerted for future reports. This dose of vitamin E, obviously, should never be used in self-medication, but it does make one wonder whether more modest supplements of the vitamin might not be a judicious practice.

Other nutritional notes on Crohn's disease are brief, as is my own experience with the disorder. In a few cases, zinc supplements have proved beneficial. This may simply have been a repair of the zinc deficiency frequent in the disorder, but it may also have invoked the healing effect of zinc, which has frequently been reported. Recovery from surgery is hastened with zinc, and the strength of stitched lesions was greater after zinc supplementation.

As with colitis, desiccated duodenal tissue has proved beneficial in ileitis. The physician familiar with this innocuous treatment gradually increases the dose of the tablets to the point where it becomes constipating, and then reduces it just below that level. Pantothenic acid therapy has proved rewarding in some patients, too.

Supplementary intake of vitamin E (mixed tocopherols) is from 200 to 400 units daily. Supplementary intake of zinc, as the gluconate or in the chelated form, is 15 mg. to 30 mg. daily. Supplementary doses of pantothenic acid are 50 mg. daily. The medical nutritionist will increase these doses by a considerable amount, and may prefer, at least initially, to administer the pantothenic acid by injection.

Since there is compelling evidence that prostaglandin E_1 is beneficial in Crohn's disease, it may be that zinc is helpful in the disorder because that metal is important in the synthesis of the prostaglandin. This would also explain why evening primrose oil has been found helpful, for it contains gamma linoleic acid, a necessary precursor for the synthesis of this hormone. This suggests that the medical nutritionist might prescribe evening primrose oil plus all the nutrients necessary to convert its gamma linoleic acid into the prostaglandin. Considering the poor utilization of nutrients likely in diseases of the digestive tract, like Crohn's, this would require supplements not only of zinc, but also of magnesium, pyridoxine (vitamin B_6), niacinamide, vitamin C, vitamin E, and, to guard against cellular oxidation of the oil, all the other antioxidants discussed in the section on arthritis.

DIABETES

Though large textbooks on diabetes crowd the shelves of medical libraries, what we really know about the disease could be condensed into a rather small monograph. Discussions of misconceptions in the public's view of diabetes would fill a fair-sized book. Ironically, some of those misconceptions are implicit in orthodox medical and dietetic management of the disorder. This I tell you so that what follows will be more acceptable to you, if nonetheless somewhat disturbing.

Though the term "diabetes" is used by the public as they use the term "arthritis"—as if each were a single disease—diabetes appears in a number of forms, several of which have not been recognized in medicine, or at least, recognition certainly isn't reflected in the treatments used. Accepted are juvenile diabetes, mature-onset diabetes (which some physicians believe to be the juvenile type, so mild that it wasn't recognized earlier), diabetes insipidus, and, recently postulated, viral diabetes. The last implies that the juvenile form results from a viral attack on the insulin-producing cells of the pancreas.

Some practitioners recognize a "geriatric" or "senile" type of diabetes, which is not full blown but does present the problem of elevation of blood glucose (sugar). Few medical professionals, other than medical nutritionists, have come to grips with the possibility that the "diabetes" of the aged may represent nothing more than the price paid for the body's inability to synthesize a glucose tolerance factor based on chromium. And only a handful of practitioners recognize the extent to which food allergy plays an important part in some cases of diabetes.

If you find it difficult to accept these omissions in medical knowledge, thinking, and practice, consider that low-carbohydrate diets were *the* diets for diabetes until a few years ago; and then, suddenly, a *high* proportion of complex carbohydrate was found for some patients to be infinitely better. Another deficit is the concept, directly reflected in what is called "management of diabetes," that control of blood glucose is control of the disease. It most certainly is not. It's an aspect of control, but incomplete, and far from satisfactory. Best proof: Some of the so-called "complications of diabetes" precede, by a considerable amount of time, elevation of blood glucose. Second proof: Mothers who show no elevation of blood sugar before or during pregnancy, and who give birth to very heavy babies (over twelve pounds) may become diabetic later. The disturbance was there, obviously, and affected the babies' prenatal weight gain; yet the mothers' blood glucose gave no hint of a diabetic process.

Not only is disturbance of carbohydrate metabolism not the whole story of diabetes, but there is evidence that the diabetic has problems with other fractions of food. For example, we normally convert vegetable vitamin A (carotene) into true vitamin A. The diabetic doesn't make the conversion and therby must depend on preformed vitamin A for his necessary supply. This difficulty is certainly not recognized in the dietary recommendations made to diabetics. In fact, what is done accomplishes the opposite: In the effort to hold down the intake of saturated fat and cholesterol, the diabetic is discouraged from eating vitamin A–rich foods like liver and eggs. The mention of fat and cholesterol brings up another metabolic error that marks the diabetic: He is prone to atherosclerosis and to heart attacks. This certainly raises questions about his body's management of fat and cholesterol.

Another misconception is reflected in the "food exchange" lists that are dispensed by every diabetologist and dietician. To the orthodox dietician, one must be a heretic to find anything wrong with food exchange lists. Yet they reflect a basic and very serious error in nutritional management of the disease. In essence, the food exchange lists encourage the diabetic, in the interests of more freedom of choice in his menus, to interchange carbohydrates of like composition and calorie value. The message is: "If you don't feel like eating spaghetti, you can choose an equal number of starch calories from rice, or exchange a given quantity of bread for a given amount of potato, or potato for corn, similarly." Behind these permitted exchanges is an assumption that is, unhappily, without foundation. In essence, the food exchange lists are based on the philosophy that starch is starch, and that, given calorie-equivalent amounts in a balanced diet, it doesn't matter which complex carbohydrate a diabetic chooses. This simply isn't so for some (and possibly many) of these patients. Starch from different sources doesn't necessarily have the same effects on the blood sugar levels of a diabetic. I am saying—on the basis not of theory, but of actual studies—that calorie-equivalent portions of rice, corn, wheat, potato, banana, and bread, as examples, will not have the same effects on blood glucose levels. Rice will raise blood glucose less than wheat, as an example. Instead of calorie-equivalent carbohydrate portions, we should be giving *biologically* equivalent portions. This truth, unfortunately, is not recognized in orthodox diabetic management. Many practitioners, in fact, don't even know that the research in this area has been done.

Diabetics are painstakingly examined when the disease strikes, but that examination rarely includes tests for allergies. Yet the diabetic, eating a food to which he is allergic—even if it isn't sugar or starch—may experience a catastrophic rise in blood sugar. I am saying explicitly that a diabetic's allergic reaction to beef or wheat, or any other such food reaction, may promote elevation in blood glucose out of all proportion to the amount and kind of the food that has been consumed.

From all this, it becomes obvious that the standard test for diabetes (which is also the test for hypoglycemia), the glucose tolerance test, is likewise based on erroneous theory. The diabetic should have a *food* tolerance test. This would not only yield the classical information about blood glucose response; it would also pick up the reactions to noncarbohydrate foods (and others) which are based on allergy. The administration of a glucose tolerance test is a statement that a diabetic's only nutrition concern is the reaction to starches and sugars. Not so.

If all this sounds like an academic tempest in a teapot, consider that there are authorities, like Michael Somogyi, who believe that some of the complications of diabetes are actually complications caused by the treatment—insulin. Even those physicians who don't accept that theory will agree that it is best to keep insulin doses as low as possible. If allergy, unrecognized as playing a role in elevating blood glucose levels, is causing the need for higher dosage of insulin, it is a service to identify the offending foods. These suggestions do not apply to insulin-dependent diabetics alone, for they may also permit lowering of the doses of the oral hypoglycemic drugs, since these drugs appear to improve the response to internally produced insulin—and an excess is undesirable, too.

The thesis that insulin is a two-edged medicine, like so many others, derives from the antagonism between adrenal hormones, which raise blood sugar, and insulin, which lowers it. When the blood glucose drops as little as 3 mg. below the level normal to the body, at a given moment, the adrenals immediately attempt to compensate. This places these glands in a continuous battle with insulin. When the source of the insulin is a hypodermic, the adrenals must, if overdose is frequent, become exhausted. At this point, the individual begins to suffer with what Dr. Hans Selye calls the "stress adaptation syndrome." If you look up the symptoms of that syndrome, you will discover, curiously, that it includes every one of the disorders that are also called the "complications of diabetes."

There are four nutritional aids to reducing requirements for insulin or hypoglycemic drugs—five, if you count reduction to normal body weight, if needed, which is always helpful. These are the chromium glucose tolerance factor, previously mentioned, desiccated liver, a specialized type of vitamin B complex supplement, and a diet emphasizing raw food and fiber.

The chromium glucose tolerance factor is synthesized in the body, combining a vitamin (niacinamide) with a complex formula that includes chromium. Deficiency in it, perhaps reflecting the aging process, possibly caused by dietary deficiencies in the precursor factors (including chromium), causes what might be called a mild diabetes, or at least, an abnormal if not dramatic rise in blood sugar. Administration of chromium itself is not helpful, the factor being useful only when it is fully preformed. The most frequently used source of the chromium glucose tolerance factor is a concentrate of it from brewer's yeast. Thus far, diabetologists have shown minimal interest in this discovery, perhaps because they think of it as being useful only in the treatment of senior citizens with mild elevation of blood sugar. Actually, medical nutritionists have found that it is useful in all types of diabetes mellitus—meaning juvenile and maturity-onset diabetes. Used properly, it may reduce the insulin requirement; in some cases, it has eliminated it. The important point to remember is the advantage a diabetic gains when he draws more upon natural aids and less upon medication.

That brings up the complications of diabetes, for which the medical armamentarium is woefully short of miracles. The hemorrhagic retinitis of diabetes, which has caused so much impairment of vision (and in some cases, blindness), is a good example. Only recently did the American Medical Association admit that vitamin E is helpful in "neovascular disease" of the eyes and in a type of cataract common in diabetics. As yet, the establishment has not recognized that the bioflavonoids are equally useful in hemorrhagic eye disease. In part, the FDA and the A.M.A. must take responsibility for this tragic and short-sighted view, for despite dozens and dozens of papers reporting usefulness of the bioflavonoids, they have persisted in denying that these substances are in any way therapeutic. But then, there is similar myopia in refusing to recognize that "sugar-free" candies and gum may be a real hazard to diabetics. These usually contain sorbitol, which is a carbohydrate more slowly absorbed than sugar, but the calorie value is the same, and sorbitol—if it escapes breakdown in the liver—can wreak havoc in the eyes, contributing directly to cataract formation.

The cultural lag cited in the Introduction obviously exists in the failure to apply to a common (and increasing) disease the benefits of harmless nutritional prevention and therapy. One would think that the orthodoxy, remembering the years in which a low-carbohydrate diet was the *only* choice for diabetes, would now ponder the fact that a high-carbohydrate (low in sugar, high in complex starches) diet has been found preferable for some patients. It has been said that medical practices are not graven in stone.

The exponents of diets high in complex carbohydrates (unprocessed whole grains) make sweeping claims that all diabetics should be so treated. I have already indicated my allergy to generalizations, and these claims should be tempered. While this type of diet has been most useful, I do know a practitioner who for years has treated some diabetics with protein accompanied by vegetable oil—with zero carbohydrate. (There are risks in that procedure, but he vows that competent supervision eliminates the difficulties, and the patients then do very well.) I am simply making the point that for some diabetics, diets high in unprocessed carbohydrate reduce their insulin requirements. Part of that benefit may accrue from the fiber in such diets, for bran has been found helpful to some diabetics. Part may derive from the chromium glucose tolerance factor, which is found in whole grains. There are also diabetics whose insulin requirements are lowered considerably by diets emphasizing raw fruits and vegetables. I do not believe that any single type of diet is *the* panacea.

Diabetic neuropathies, another "complication of diabetes" are a glittering example of the failure to practice prevention in place of crisis medicine. These are disorders of the nervous system, usually involving the lower part of the body and causing a woeful array of symptoms, ranging from chronic pain in the legs to diarrhea, gas pains, and constipation, from circulatory problems to sexual impotence. A recent report confirms what I learned many years ago, in research with Dr. Wolfgang Seligmann: If you give vitamin B complex in high enough doses to diabetics with nervous system disturbances, you reduce their pain and help to normalize the disturbances of motor and sensory function. The report deals only with vitamin B_{12}, given in doses (by injection) of 50 mg. daily, plus 200 mg. of B_6 and 300 mg. of B_1. There are two deficits in that recital: Other B vitamins affect the nervous system, and within the limitations of those available for injection, they should have been administered, too. This would, for instance, include niacinamide, pantothenate, folic acid, inositol, and choline. Second, and even more important: Why wait until a diabetic develops neuropathies? Why not give all insulin-dependent diabetics prophylactic doses of the vitamins, by mouth, from the day the disorder is diagnosed? Does it smack too much of prevention?

The last of the misconceptions about diabetes is the belief that the misbehaving pancreas (or resistance to insulin) is *the* explanation for the disease. Not so; in animals, one can tie off the pancreas, administer sugar and a little insulin, and the liver will maintain normal blood glucose levels. But if you reverse that—if you interfere with liver function *and* administer sugar, the pancreas will not normally control blood glucose levels.

Back in the 1930s, when physicians were alarmed by side reactions to insulin, they sought alternate and safer methods of treatment. They found that supplements of liver normalized blood glucose levels with such efficiency that they published a monograph indicating exactly how much liver was needed to offset a given dose of insulin. That report, like so many others invoking nutrition as a substitute for medication, was ignored. When I discovered it, I suggested to an internist that treatment aimed at normalizing liver function might be useful to diabetics. This suggested the use of a vitamin B complex concentrate high in such lipotropic factors as choline and inositol. (This was decades before inositol was recognized as helpful in normalizing nerve transmission in diabetics—but this is another report that was ignored.) When we encountered an obese diabetic who was allergic to insulin, and who was unwilling to reduce or to eat a controlled diet, we supplemented her ill-chosen meals with the vitamin concentrate, and in sixteen weeks her blood glucose dropped more than 100 mg.—not to normal, but much closer to it; her vision improved from 3-300 to 3-25, and her urine, 4+ for sugar when we started, was normal at the sixteenth week. All this with great obesity and no dietary control.

Considering the reported benefits of liver for diabetics, and the dividends from vitamin B complex therapy for diabetic neuropathies, one could conservatively conclude that there are compelling reasons to give every diabetic the possible dividends of such reenforcement, from day one of the diagnosis, or even earlier. For patients not yet diabetics, but generally susceptible to the disease or with glucose tolerance tests not fully normal, the B complex may prove a great boon.

DISORDERS OF MIND AND MOOD

A relatively minor deficiency in thiamine for a few months will make you hostile, asocial, aggressive, and unable to concentrate. With a chronic, mild deficiency in niacinamide, you hear voices that are not there, are distracted by minor noises, and have horrible nightmares, which awaken you from sleep, dripping in perspiration; but with a severe deficiency, you will be completely psychotic. Lack of vitamin B_6 (pyridoxine) will make dream recall difficult and short-term memory unreliable. It will also help to distort reality for the autistic. These are not theories, but part of our hard-won knowledge of the chemistry of nutrition in mind and mood.

The orthodoxy in psychiatry continues to neglect the helpfulness of nutrition in mental and emotional disorders. It is more than neglect; it is active and irrational hostility. Just as it is important for you to understand the brainwashing that orthodox medicine inflicted on physicians who might otherwise be diagnosing and treating hypoglycemia, so it is urgent that you know why the average psychiatrist and psychoanalyst regards orthomolecular psychiatry as quackery. In part the attitude was created originally by the American Psychiatric Association, which reported to the professions and the public that it had tested vitamin therapy in schizophrenia and found it utterly useless. The background for that pronouncement is fascinating. The research was performed by a committee headed by a psychiatrist who admitted that, before even beginning the experiment, he was prejudiced against nutritional treatment for schizophrenia. A second member of the committee said that he wouldn't believe in orthomolecular treatment even if *every* psychiatrist in America told him that it was effective. A third member, it was reported, had been on the payroll of a tranquilizer manufacturer. With such a committee, the manner in which the experiment was conducted should not have been unexpected. They used one vitamin—niacinamide—on hospitalized schizophrenics and witnessed not one single benefit in one year of treatment of 1,000 patients. But those who pioneered in vitamin therapy for schizophrenics long ago warned physicians that niacinamide alone has no effect on chronic, advanced schizophrenia, helping only early, mild cases. By definition, hospitalized schizophrenics are anything but early, mild cases. Despite the obvious built-in bias in the test, its results were widely quoted as "proving" that orthomolecular psychiatry is a snare and a delusion. But exactly as the A.M.A. insisted that hypoglycemia was imaginary, and then gave a course in diagnosis and treatment of it, so did the authorities in psychiatry condemn orthomolecular therapy, while simultaneously asking the Academy of Orthomolecular Psychiatry for a referral list of such practitioners, for the benefit of patients wishing to consult them. (I should note that I am not writing merely as an exterior observer of this scene, since I am an honorary fellow of that academy.) It will occur to the unbiased that psychiatrists who prescribe drugs such as tranquilizers and antidepressants should philosophically be amenable to nutritional therapies aimed at the same targets—the nervous systems and the brain; logic, though, has not been a characteristic of the opposition to the harmless therapies, though one would think they would be seized on, for the profession prescribing tranquilizers has found it necessary to create clinics for the sole purpose of treating side reactions to these medications. I tell you all this so that you aren't blocked in seeking nutritional help for mental and emotional problems.

Depression

You may be depressed because your genes dictate such a brain chemistry. If it runs in your family, your depression is not related to your life situation, and represents the end product of disturbed chemistry of thinking and emotions. You may be depressed because of the wrong job, the wrong spouse, or the anguish of catastrophic disasters in your life. Dictation by the genes isn't a prerequisite to disturbance of brain chemistry, but—and this is the important point—without that disturbance, there will be no depression. Orthodox treatment with drugs and orthomolecular treatment, although using very different agents, are both directed to the chemistry of thinking and feeling. The drug hides the symptoms; the nutrients often remove the cause.

In both sexes, depression may be caused by food intolerances that affect brain function. Such sensitivities can be identified and the offending foods (or drugs, or chemicals) removed from the environment. Don't discount this. Long ago, I told the story of a little girl who, subjected to inhaling Lysol spray, took electric light bulbs from ceiling fixtures in the allergist's office and dropped them into the waste basket, explaining that she was planting seeds in her garden. Given a neutralizing dose of pyridoxine and vitamin C, she returned to normal, but could remember nothing of her behavior. During the attack, she addressed her mother by the name of a male teacher she had had three years before, and described the allergist as yellow dots on a purple background. The case is cited so that you may realize that depression would be a mild expression of this process. So would anxiety.

Traditional allergists are not comfortable with the concept of cerebral allergy. Exactly why would require pages for a complete explanation, but suffice it to say that their definition of allergy demands a certain type of reaction from the immune system (IgE or immungobulin E). Failing such evidence, they will not themselves term it allergy. It would seem to be an academic tempest, but it prevents them from recognizing mental and emotional disturbances that can originate with intolerance for foods, chemicals, and drugs. The bioecological allergists are a different breed. They know from experience that allergy to hydrocarbons can make your new plastic tiling the source of inexplicable depression, or automobile exhaust the reason for anxiety you suddenly develop on long automobile trips. It has been suggested that we drop the term "cerebral allergy" and call it "maladaptive reaction." The orthodox allergists may feel more comfortable with this term, since it seems to cover a "new" type of reaction.

In women, depression may be triggered during the premenstrual week, when hormone activity elevates the copper levels in the blood. The same effect might be anticipated in some pregnancies and in the use of the birth control pill, and for exactly the same reason: hormone influence in raising blood copper levels. Excess copper may also be carried to you by drinking water, particularly if it is soft water and conveyed by the copper piping so widely used. Other causes of high blood copper levels, causing depression, are supplements supplying excess copper, chronic stress or inflammation, or dietary deficiencies in copper antagonists, such as zinc, manganese, or molybdenum. In addition to causing depression, copper toxicity can also be responsible for painful joints, hypertension, premature baldness, tinnitus (ringing in the ears), facial pigmentation, and insomnia.

For depression so caused, orthomolecular treatment starts by decreasing copper supplies, if possible. Where drinking water is the offender, a shift to bottled beverage water may be the only remedy. Supplements of zinc, manganese, or molybdenum, or a combination of these, may be used, with vitamin C, to bring down the copper levels by increasing excretion of the metal. In resistant cases, a chelating agent such as penicillamine may be used. Ordinarily a drug with intolerable side reactions, this medication becomes better tolerated when given in a low dose. Its use must be accompanied with vitamin B_6 and zinc—the vitamin to help the absorption of the zinc, and the zinc because it is an effective copper antagonist.

This is not a therapy for self-medicators. Dosage is critical, and there are sometimes complications that necessitate a change in dosage. For example, as copper is removed from the blood, the supply in the tissues may move to the blood. This will cause a temporary elevation rather than a drop in blood copper, and symptoms may for a short time worsen. At that point, the competent physician will lower the zinc dose to slow the process, and subsequently raise it. About three months of treatment will be needed for the maximum improvement.

The peculiarities of the biochemistry of some people make them prone to copper accumulation, for which constant supplements of vitamin C and zinc must be used. Therapeutic dose information will be supplied to your physician on request. The amount of zinc and manganese in diet supplements may not be adequate to combat elevated copper. Molybdenum is not usually provided in such supplements. Vitamin C, of course, can be taken in the usual range of supplementary dose: 250 mg. to 2,500 mg. daily.

In the section on hypoglycemia, I report that of the patients with hypoglycemia studied by a physician expert in managing the disorder, 20 percent reported depression to a suicidal degree. This obviously means that patients with depression, particularly when it is suicidal, should be tested for low blood sugar. The symptoms disappear almost magically when hypoglycemia is corrected.

Elevated blood histamine has been identified as the cause of a type of schizophrenia in which suicidal depression is a constant threat. This type of schizophrenia doesn't respond to any of the usual drug therapies, shock treatment, or the classical megavitamin therapy for schizophrenia, as developed by Abram Hoffer and Humphrey Osmund. I am aware that my readers are not likely to be schizophrenics, but I have a good reason to ask you, if you are depressed, to consider the possibility that the disturbed chemistry of this psychosis may cause depression in nonschizophrenic and otherwise normal individuals.

Since the various biochemical types of schizophrenia are described in the following subsection, I am interested here only in the possibility that the nutritional therapy used for the high-histamine type might be applicable to depression in mentally normal individuals who have elevated histamine levels. A description of such therapy is included in the discussion of the schizophrenias. It often relieves their depression in a month or less. Since allergic persons often have significantly elevated histamine levels, the same treatment has been beneficial to them, too. This is important, not only for relief from many allergy symptoms, but because allergy itself can cause depression, just as it can trigger explosive outbursts of rage alien to the normal personality, and irritability, and a host of other "emotional" and "mental" symptoms. To appreciate the importance of what I am saying about allergy as a factor in depression, consider the case of a woman who was under psychoanalysis and drug treatment for depression for a period of several years, when a bioecological allergist discovered that her problem came from sensitivity to the chlorine in drinking water. She thereafter stayed depression-free by the simple device of carrying her own spring water with her, but was thrown into despair when a profound depression followed a social evening where, she insisted, she had not consumed the hostess's drinking water. She hadn't—but she had used her ice cubes, and that was enough of a chlorine source to disturb her brain chemistry.

In the treatment of Parkinson's syndrome (see page 150) an amino acid, phenylalanine, proved markedly beneficial in relieving the depression common in that disorder. It doesn't matter whether the depression is part of the disease or is caused by the emotional reaction to a progressive and crippling disorder. In either case, the amino acid necessarily must have had a beneficial effect on a neurotransmitter in the brain, or on its modulators in the cells. To my knowledge, there have been no controlled studies of the effect of the protein on depression in individuals who do not have Parkinson's, but one would certainly be justified.

When depression is of internal origin—that is, not related to the life situation—neither antidepressant drugs nor psychotherapy should be the first therapy. The possibility of a genetic factor should be investigated. Recently, a family with a history of suicides in three generations was investigated. A third-generation survivor, also suicidal, was found to have low brain serotonin levels. Similarly low levels of this neurotransmitter were found on autopsy of a recent suicide in that family. Serotonin is a "quieting" neurotransmitter. A deficit in it can have profound effects on brain function, cognition, and moods. Yet it is possible to raise serotonin levels with tryptophane (an amino acid), pyridoxine (vitamin B_6), and niacinamide.

Hydrocarbon sensitivity is a frequent cause of disturbances previously thought to be purely emotional. An orthomolecular practitioner tells the story of a woman who moved into a house inherited from her mother and suffered devastating depression, apparently coming out of the blue, for several years. She was forced into psychoanalysis, which may have benefited the practitioner, but did nothing for her. A fortuitous choice of a dinner guest led to her recovery. He noticed the odor of gasoline in the house, which, she explained, came from a car parked in a garage under the home. When she moved the car to the driveway, part of her depression left. The rest disappeared when she reluctantly consented to remove the plastic tiling in her kitchen. The plastic was of petroleum origin.

If one is wedded to psychoanalysis or other psychiatric therapy, there is no collision between the couch and the nutritional therapies. In fact, there is compelling evidence that good diet and appropriate vitamin, mineral, and amino acid therapy will improve the response to psychiatric treatment, making it easier for the patient to communicate with the practitioner. I am addressed, though, to a situation that is all too common: when the patient, whose problem is hypoglycemia, elevated copper, high histamine, or a neurotransmitter imbalance, is conversationally dredging up emotional insults from childhood as the sole effort to obtain relief. Or even worse: swallowing drugs with more penalties than dividends.

The Schizophrenias

I recall a psychiatrist, one of the staff in a state mental hospital, telling an anguished father whose schizophrenic daughter had just been carried away, screaming, in restraint, that he must have been too busy in his occupation to pay necessary attention to the girl in her formative years. As the "healer" for a disease he can't heal and doesn't understand, this practitioner was adding undeserved guilt to the burden of a distraught father. Let's begin, then, with two truths: Conversation and the couch have never helped schizophrenics fully to recover, and there is evidence that some harm has been the sole dividend. Second, the drug therapies for schizophrenia may quiet the "voices" they hear, calm aggressive behavior, and make the patients manageable—to be turned out into society with their disease still full blown, as sick as ever they were. Moreover, as I remarked earlier, the neuroleptic drugs that achieve these "benefits" (surely an ill-chosen description) have side reactions which can be irreversible and which occur so frequently that clinics have been organized for the sole purpose of treating the fragmented involuntary movements of these victims of the drug culture. The disorder is called "tardive dyskinesia." If you detect more than a note of indignation in this writing, it is because I know of a single orthomolecular psychiatric clinic that has treated some 10,000 schizophrenics without a single case of tardive dyskinesia—even in those whose treatment combined nutritional therapies *and* drugs. If the use of the drugs in an orthomolecular institution strikes you as contradictory, let me disabuse you of that thought. When a schizophrenic has been brought back to a reality he has not perceived for years, it may be helpful to augment the nutritional treatment with mild doses of the tranquilizers and antipsychosis drugs, to help him to bridge the first few difficult weeks or months.

Another ironic note is the establishment's treatment for tardive dyskinesia. They have discovered the usefulness of lecithin—a supplement we nutritionists and the orthomolecular practitioners have been using for decades. They have not yet discovered that manganese is helpful too, for the same reason that it aids some epileptics.

In addition to the error of considering various types of schizophrenia as being facets of a single disease, the psychiatric establishment has been guilty of using what I should call the modern equivalent of the snake pit into which the insane were thrown, in a medieval attempt to dispossess the demons supposed to be causing the illness.

This is shock therapy (or ECT, electroconvulsive therapy). If you ask why it is occasionally helpful, you will be told no one knows, for the only visible effect (observable on autopsy) is small, punctuate hemorrhages in the brain. One of the side benefits claimed for the treatment, which is primarily aimed against depression, is relief from allergies. It has not yet occurred to the psychiatrists that they may be relieving *brain* allergy, which is a very potent factor in the troubles of a majority of schizophrenics. But then, the psychiatrists don't recognize brain allergy, and think the bioecological allergists and orthomolecular practitioners who do identify and treat it are exploiting uninformed patients.

With all this, those who are competent in nutritional treatment for schizophrenia have identified three biochemical models of the disorder, all different; and there are probably a half-hundred more. Writing with the assumption that you are reading this because schizophrenia is a problem for you, a member of your family, or a friend, I am going to outline what orthomolecular psychiatry has learned about this group of diseases. You may well find help for the patient in what follows. There is comfort in the realization that tens of thousands of schizophrenics have been restored to sanity by these harmless treatments. That record is even more impressive when you realize that the patients who come to orthomolecular practitioners and institutions are the *failures* of the orthodox therapies.

Schizophrenia is a disease of perception, with inability to judge whether the changes are real. There is thought disorder, great fatigue, and marked depression. Early, mild cases have been treated successfully with vitamin B_3—niacinamide. Generally, the vitamin is given in the niacinamide form until nausea sets in, which may be at doses over 2 or 2.5 g., and the practitioner then completes the dose by using niacin, which is the form of the vitamin that causes flushing. Don't discount this treatment, however simplistic it sounds. It has rescued many schizophrenics, and I write that as one who has had the opportunity to observe the treatment and its results. Vitamin C is also given to many patients, and proves helpful. The sicker the schizophrenic is, the less of the vitamin C he will excrete in the urine, even when the dose is so large that the body, ordinarily, would part with most of it. As the patient improves, the vitamin C excretion increases, and it is theoretically possible to appraise the progress of a schizophrenic one has never seen, merely by examining, day by day, the amount of vitamin C excreted in his urine. Vitamin B_6 benefits many schizophrenics, and doses are large. Vitamin E is useful to some of these patients.

We have been discussing schizophrenia in general terms. Let me now take you through a brief study of three different biochemical models of schizophrenia, identified through the pioneering research of Dr. Carl C. Pfeiffer of the Brain Bio Center in Princeton, New Jersey. The first is the high-histamine schizophrenic. Histamine is a neurotransmitter, with many functions in the body at large, as well as the brain. Excessive histamine activity in schizophrenia is associated with persistent thoughts of suicide, and these patients must constantly be guarded against self-destruction. The depression is accompanied by twisted perceptions of reality and by compulsions, thought disorder, abnormal fears, feelings of confusion, a blank mind, and easy crying. Addictions to drugs are common in this type of schizophrenia. Conversely, high histamine levels are found in many drug addicts (not schizophrenic), offering the possibility that the treatment found helpful in such schizophrenics might be useful for the addicts. Allergies and cyclical headaches are common. Tolerance for pain is extremely low, and insomnia, that twin sister to depression, is a severe problem. These patients can—without going to sleep as a result—take doses of sleeping drugs that could be dangerous or even lethal for a normal person. One of the consequences of the biochemical disturbance in high-histamine schizophrenics is an intolerance for folic acid, meaning not only doses of the concentrated vitamin, but even the relatively small amount in a large green salad. For these people, folic acid increases depression.

Because of the folic acid intolerance, it was logical to try a drug—Dilantin—ordinarily used for epilepsy, which has an anti–folic acid action. (This explains some of the side reactions of Dilantin when epileptics take the drug for long periods.) For the high-histamine schizophrenic, Dilantin is used in small doses. Vitamin B_{12}, which may reduce the level of depression, is well tolerated. Calcium, methionine (an amino acid that helps to reduce histamine levels), zinc, and manganese are used, since the minerals also have an antihistamine effect. This therapy will often relieve depression in the high-histamine schizophrenics in a month or less, but much longer treatment is needed for the obsessions, rituals, and phobias. If treatment is stopped, symptoms return.

Since allergy patients often have elevated histamine levels, it is logical that the same treatment has been found beneficial in that disorder. This is important, not only for the relief of allergy, but because allergy itself can cause depression, irritability, uncontrollable rage, and a host of other symptoms. One must wonder, in the light of research with the high-histamine schizophrenics, whether the elevated level of histamine involved in allergy may be directly responsible for some of these symptoms. While we're wondering, we might speculate that people with confused thinking, blank minds, and feelings of confusion, who do *not* have schizophrenia, may nonetheless be victims of high histamine too.

The treatment for all schizophrenias must, obviously, be medically supervised. If your physician wishes guidance, he can communicate with the Brain Bio Center. (See the Appendix for the address.)

The possibility of prevention was suggested by research initiated by Dr. Linus Pauling. It was predicated on the observation that very sick schizophrenics retain doses of vitamin C that normal people would largely excrete. The research proposed administration of substantial doses of vitamin C, vitamin B_6, and niacinamide to children, and measurement of the amounts excreted; the thesis being that the child retaining unusually large percentages of the vitamins would be most in danger. The thesis has never been investigated, and obviously should be, for children in families with a history of schizophrenia, if for no one else. Another hint of possible prevention—not applicable to all schizophrenics nor to all types of the disease— would be elimination of wheat from the diet. The disease is rare in rice-eating countries, and wheat gluten (protein) is known to worsen the disorder in a substantial percentage of schizophrenics. Wartime blockades that deprived Europeans of wheat contributed to a sharp drop in admissions to mental hospitals for treatment of schizophrenia. Which doesn't explain why bread remains a staple in mental hospital menus, does it? One doesn't avoid wheat, which is for most of us a good food, arbitrarily. There are sensitive tests for such intolerance (see Allergies). Apropos of food tolerance, these patients do badly on a high-protein diet.

A second type of schizophrenia is pyrroluria. The name signifies the presence in the blood of a substance—kryptopyrrole, which has a property of combining with vitamin B_6 first, and then with zinc, thereby taking both out of the body. Histamine levels are normal. As the niacinamide and vitamin C treatment helpful in another type of schizophrenia does not benefit high-histamine patients, so will neither of these treatments help the kryptopyrrole group. Their symptoms include chronic insomnia, loss of contact with reality occurring at intervals, suicidal depression, loss of memory, partial seizures (convulsions), nausea, vomiting, and cessation of the menses. The breath is abnormally sweet, and the skin may be excessively sensitive to sunshine. Cartilage and tendon development is abnormal because of the lack of vitamin B_6 and zinc, deficiencies that have the same effect in lower animals. There are disturbances of the bone marrow, with resulting anemia, which is also caused by the deficiencies. Adverse reactions to tranquilizers and barbiturates result from the deficiency in enzymes needed to detoxify these drugs, again because of the vitamin-mineral deficiency. Recall of dreams is poor or nonexistent. Spasms of the muscles may be so violent as to require restraint.

What happens to a victim of pyrroluria when the cause is not recognized? Actual case histories tell us: years of drugs that are not tolerated; years of psychotherapy that is ineffective; even shock treatment. They are labeled paranoid schizophrenics, or other variations on the theme, and they deteriorate in institutions. As for the attitude of the orthodox psychiatrist toward a biochemical approach to this, actually a problem in disturbed biochemistry, there is on record a psychiatrist who objected because the vitamin B_6 changed dreams from nightmares to pleasant ones. Nightmares, he insisted, were useful for elimination of inner aggression, and the shift to pleasant dreams was thereby not progress, but a step backward.

Pyrroluric patients by the thousands have been treated successfully with this simple therapy, vitamin B_6, manganese, and zinc, at some twenty clinics and three brain bio centers. Of interest is the instruction they receive to increase their already large doses of the vitamin and the mineral whenever they are under stress. Perhaps it will give you pause for thought if you picture a dinner party where a guest excuses himself, telling his hostess that he is a diabetic and must take his insulin injection. While not an eyebrow would rise with this pronouncement, consider what would happen if the guest said he was a pyrroluric and must take his zinc and pyridoxine to preserve his physical and mental well-being. Yet, scientifically speaking, the situations are the same, for the insulin and the vitamin and the minerals all represent supplements some people need.

The third type of schizophrenia is the opposite of the high histamine. These patients have low histamine and abnormally high blood copper levels. They are less depressed than the high-histamine group, suffer less from a "blank mind," complain much more of thought disorder and delusions of persecution. They are more subject to hallucinations and less troubled by obsessions and phobias. These patients show an excellent response to treatment with niacin and vitamin C. Their reaction to folic acid—which disturbs the high-histamine schizophrenic—is excellent and, sometimes, dramatic. The high-protein diet, which isn't helpful to high-histamine patients, is excellent for the low-histamine group. These patients also have a better reaction to shock therapy. Zinc and manganese therapy benefit them, though somewhat less than the high-histamine group. Dilantin makes them worse, which one would anticipate, considering their favorable response to folic acid.

About 60 percent of the schizophrenics tested for hypoglycemia prove to be victims of it. This doesn't mean their troubles were caused by low blood sugar, but you can be certain that hypoglycemia will make those symptoms worse. These people should of course be placed on the diet for low blood sugar (see Hypoglycemia). If this yields no other dividend, and it *will*—it will make the patient more responsive to all the other therapies.

Often I receive pleading letters from patients or relatives of patients in the wilds of Alaska or Africa, or even in metropolitan areas of large cities here and abroad, who are unable to find a practitioner willing to entertain alternatives to the couch, conversation, calmative drugs, and shock therapy. They wish, as you yourself might in such circumstances, to be directed in applying nutritional therapies to psychosis. There is no way in which fair treatment of people so sick can be managed by the layman. It must be obvious from what you have read that thorough testing must precede therapy, encompassing hair, blood, and urine analyses. However, all you need is a modicum of cooperation from your physician—better he than an indoctrinated and resistant orthodox psychiatrist—and he can obtain the information he needs from the agencies listed in the Appendix of this book.

Prevention is another matter. To give you an idea of the value of a balanced diet, coupled with a nontherapeutic multiple vitamin-mineral supplement, just reflect on the penalties for zinc deficiency, which you must now appreciate, and realize that the zinc value of the American diet is so marginal that a single day of total fasting may cause the white spots of zinc deficiency to appear—later, of course—

in the fingernails. If there is a history of schizophrenia in the family, the need for expert testing and treatment becomes, of course, more urgent. The mention of family history should not lead you astray. Adolescence often brings with it emotional disturbances that ordinarily may be nothing more than the tug of war between the desire to mature and the fear of leaving the protected sanctuary of childhood.

My prime purpose in this discussion should be obvious. I have watched with anguish the toll of schizophrenia, not only on the patient, but on the family. Some of these patients *can* escape the snake pit.

DISTURBANCES OF SMELL AND TASTE

It is often early in pregnancy that many women find familiar foods distasteful and familiar odors unbearable. In that stage of pregnancy, the baby is beginning to draw upon the mother's zinc reserves, which, if she eats like the average American, are so limited that a single day of fasting may deplete them enough to cause a white spot to develop later on the nails.

This is one of the bits of evidence that point to zinc as a factor needed to support the senses of smell and taste. Another is found in the loss of both faculties when one has been dosed with antibiotics. This is usually blamed on the cold which is being treated, but it may derive from a chelating action of the antibiotics, which would promote the excretion of zinc. The deficiency may, instead of diminishing the senses of taste and smell, distort them, so that ordinarily acceptable (or even accustomed) tastes and odors become disgusting.

It isn't zinc alone that is needed to support these faculties. Vitamin A is related, in ways we do not yet understand. Vitamin B_6 (pyridoxine) intake is also important, because in the absence of an adequate supply of this vitamin, zinc absorption is impaired.

For all these reasons, supplements of zinc, vitamin A, and vitamin B_6 are employed to try to help those whose senses of smell and taste are distorted or depreciated, in the absence of any disease to explain the phenomenon. Supplementary amounts will be label doses—15 mg. to 30 mg. of zinc, as the gluconate, daily; 10,000 units of vitamin A; 10 mg. to 25 mg. of vitamin B_6. Once again, the medical nutritionist may increase these doses.

DREAMS: THOSE YOU CAN'T REMEMBER, THOSE YOU WANT TO FORGET

Inability to remember dreams may seem inconsequential until your psychoanalyst accuses you of refusing to do your homework and your nutritionist advises you that dream recall is part of short-term memory. All this offers the possibility that stimulating recall of dreams may sharpen short-term memory.

We picked up the clue to the putative role of nutrition in dream recall from research with schizophrenics of the type who respond to treatment with vitamin B_6, zinc, and manganese. (This is the type suffering with pyrroluria—see page 51.) Recall of dreams in such schizophrenics is virtually nil until they begin to take vitamin B_6. As the dose of the vitamin is increased, their dreams become more and more vivid, and recall then improves. If the dose becomes too high, the dreams may seem so real as to awaken them from sleep, which becomes the clue to the need to reduce the intake. We start them with hundreds of milligrams of vitamin B_6 daily, since this is therapy, and may go as high as 2,000 mg. per day, particularly in periods when they are under stress. For dream recall in normal individuals, supplementary amounts of the vitamin may be sufficient—from 10 mg. to 25 mg. daily.

When dreams become nightmares, poor nutrition may be the culprit. Chronic mild deficiency in thiamine (vitamin B_1) may have this effect—more so with the mild, persistent deficiency than with the acute one. A chronic deficiency in niacinamide will also bring terrors into your nights. By terrors, I mean not only nightmares, but night terror, which is a different phenomenon. Supplementary amounts of these vitamins, meaning label dosage, may be adequate to over-come mild deficiencies, though the medical nutritionist often will begin with much higher amounts.

DRUG AND ALCOHOL DETOXIFICATION

Addicts to alcohol or drugs will frequently remark that they've been through "detox" a dozen times. The need for repeated treatment points to the failure to rehabilitate the addict to the point where he no longer has the craving. The thrust of the orthodox agencies is not in that direction. Their efforts are aimed at drying out the alcoholic or, with the drug addict, arriving at the point where blood and urine no longer show evidence of drug use. When the alcoholic has dried out and is eating regularly, he may or may not receive counseling, but he will probably be referred to Alcoholics Anonymous. When the drug addict is off the drugs, has gone through the withdrawal symp-toms, and has or has not received counseling, he, too, is released. Yet, given an escape from the cultural lag in which nutrition has long been captive, there is a great deal more that can be done for ad-dicts. That "great deal more" consists not only of freeing them from the habit.

We are not talking about esoteric nutritional therapies. We are dealing—we *must* deal—with the neglected fact that these addicts have two problems. One is the use of the drug; the second is pro-found malnourishment, which can't be remedied with three meals, however "good," daily. The alcoholic is malnourished because he has substituted liquor for food; the drug addict, because both the drug effects and the pursuit of funds to feed the habit leave little incentive and less money to feed the body. If that malnourishment is not treated, it doesn't make any difference how often the addict is detoxified. It is a fundamental axiom in nutrition that long-continued malnourishment requires nutritional therapy that goes far beyond three meals daily. It must be concentrated nutritional therapy; it must be consistent; and it must be continued.

The coffee-and-doughnut offering to alcoholics is traditional.

There are five teaspoonfuls of sugar in a doughnut and usually added sugar in the coffee. If you have read the explanation of hypoglycemia in this book, you now know that sugar and caffeine worsen low blood sugar. Every true alcoholic is hypogylcemic, but in a sizable percentage of the cases, the low blood sugar *precedes* the alcoholism, and actually causes it. In short, as the average hypoglycemic craves sweets, the alcoholic twists the craving into an appetite for liquor. If he was driven into his habit by low blood sugar, the doughnuts and coffee will stimulate the process that made him an alcoholic. Nor is it irrelevant that animals addicted to alcohol will increase their intake when fed caffeine!

When you discuss this with the establishment in the field, they don't hear what you're saying. "We know!" is the response. "All alcoholics become hypoglycemic." Which is not what we are saying. This isn't academic, for the hypoglycemic who has become an alcoholic can be cured of the second condition by controlling the first one.

Therapeutic doses of niacinamide by mouth and sodium ascorbate (vitamin C) by vein have vastly benefited alcoholics. One of the founders of Alcoholics Anonymous was impressed by the results of orthomolecular therapy of this type for these addicts, indicating that niacinamide treatment greatly accelerated the responses of alcoholics to all other treatment, including psychiatric therapy. With vitamin C, in a drug addict project in California for which I am an adivser, astonishing results have been obtained when detoxification was augmented with treatment of underlying nutritional deficiencies—particularly in protein. This, the Rio Hondo Area Drug Project, has demonstrated not only much faster detoxification of both drug and alcohol addicts, but two other, very important dividends: The patients lose their craving, and if they experimentally try the addictive substance, there is no "high." Thus far, to my knowledge, the people who run this project have had no failures, though they may of course encounter some. And thus far, what they are doing has studiously been ignored by the establishments in the field.

The hypoglycemia diet represents nothing more than good nutrition, and can be applied to any addict able to tolerate frequent, small meals with restricted simple carbohydrates and adequate fat and protein. Even modest supplementing helps these sufferers. Injections of vitamins are needed, and will speed the process, but oral doses of vitamins and minerals at supplementary levels will be helpful, too. These include vitamin C (as sodium ascorbate), 250 mg. to 2,500 mg. daily; multiple vitamins and multiple minerals; and a B-complex concentrate, augmented with added niacinamide, 100 mg. daily. The protein-rich prebreakfast drink recommended with the hypoglycemia diet is useful.

Other nutritional treatment for drug and alcohol addicts will depend on the results of a test for blood histamine levels. In one series of such analyses, *all* addicts proved to have high histamine levels, leading the investigator to conclude that this abnormality, with its impact on the brain function, is probably a major force in creating addiction. If histamine is elevated, the addict must also receive the treatment described for schizophrenics of this type, as discussed on page 49.

DRY EYES

Lack of sufficient flow of tears is an obvious impediment to wearing contact lenses. When this is not a symptom of a systemic disorder, such as Sjögren's syndrome, a simple nutritional aid may solve the problem. In a number of cases reported in Canadian research, a daily supplement of 500 mg. of pyridoxine (vitamine B_6) has increased tearing sufficiently to allow the wearing of lenses.

Again in the absence of systemic disease, when there is no response or an inadequate response to the vitamin, there is a much more complex nutritional approach that is sometimes helpful. I believe that the effect of vitamin B_6 derives from its action as a precursor of the synthesis in the body of a prostaglandin—E_1—and hold the hormone responsible for the effect on eye moisture. However, vitamin B_6 deficiency is not the only one that interferes with the manufacture of the prostaglandin in the body. Also needed are niacinamide, ascorbic acid (vitamin C), zinc, and magnesium. Then there are factors that interfere with the synthesis of the hormone. These include lack of insulin, excessive intake of alcohol, excessive intake of animal fats, excessive intake of trans fats, and failure of the aging body to complete one of the essential steps in the manufacture of the hormone.

One will need a medical nutritionist to set therapeutic doses of niacinamide, vitamin C, zinc, vitamin E, vitamin B_6 and magnesium. Label dosage will set the supplementary level, which has been cited repeatedly earlier in this book. The magnesium requirement, which is usually the ceiling for magnesium used as a supplement, is 400 mg., but therapeutic doses are higher.

Trans fats, to answer the question raised a paragraph ago, are formed when fats are partially hydrogenated. On page 164 you will find a discussion of their impact in some common human disorders.

EPILEPSY

I regard the conventional medical treatment for the epilepsies as malpractice, not only for what is being done, but for what is omitted. The best way to tell you the story is to review the history of a little girl with epilepsy who was fortunate because her mother refused to surrender to the toll of the drugs with which the child was saturated.

Until she was a little over two years of age, the child was normal, bright, alert. Suddenly, without provocation of any kind, she began to have seizures, which were diagnosed as petit mal epilepsy. This was based on examination of the brain waves, for a brain scan revealed no structural abnormality. In the absence of such a physical anomaly, the child was promptly dosed with a large amount of phenobarbital, and when that failed, with an array of antiepilepsy drugs. Three years of this converted her into a near-vegetable—obese, lethargic, withdrawn, and, as the mother was told by a school for "special children," retarded and largely ineducable. Keep in mind that this was a bright, normal, little girl before the parade of medication, which not only didn't help her, but at least allowed (if not caused) her epileptic condition to become worse, for now she developed the major convulsions, or grand mal epilepsy—invariably on awakening, and usually after meals. The last phrase is a clue. It was ignored by her physicians.

The child had become so uncoordinated that she constantly bumped into furniture, constantly fell, and routinely hurt herself. The mother attributed much of this to the medication, but how does one stop treatment that is supposed to be protecting an epileptic child? She found the escape through a newspaper article telling the story of another little girl, similarly epileptic, who had been helped to escape drugs and epilepsy thanks to the treatment given by a medical nutritionist, whom she promptly tracked down by telephoning the other child's mother. She discovered to her delight that the doctor mentioned in the article practiced in the city in which she herself lived.

The child was examined for heavy metal poisoning, for metabolic abnormalities, and for nutritional deficiencies. No metal toxicity was found, but a number of nutrient deficiencies were identified, and several metabolic abnormalities resulting from them. She was then treated for food allergies. As so frequently it happens, she reacted violently to a number of the foods of which she was most fond. This is characteristic in cerebral allergy, in a process similar to that of drug addiction. The drug is taken not only for the "high" but for protection against withdrawal effects; so with the food—eating it makes the allergy-addicted feel better, and it avoids the withdrawal effects, which are very real.

The child was given a rotation diet, which excluded foods that were sensitizing for her. In such a diet, menus are arranged so that a given food—beef, for example—is the sole protein for an entire day, but is not repeated for four, five, or six days; thus, a rotation diet shifts vegetables and fruits, grains, and other foods, day by day, giving the body a chance to erect defenses. To this were added concentrates of the nutrients in which she was deficient. With this therapy, the petit mal attacks, which had been frequent, disappeared, but the grand mal episodes did not. At this point, the physician decided that the child had a problem in utilizing vitamin B_6, based on her enzyme chemistries, and gave her a sulfur-containing amino acid, cystine, in an effort to stimulate production of an enzyme indispensable in the body's utilization of vitamin B_6. A week later, the grand mal attacks stopped. In three months, the "retarded" little girl was her bright and alert self, interested in everything a little girl finds interesting, and catching up with all the activities she had missed between the ages of two and five. Said the physician: "A cause can be determined for fifty percent of the epilepsies. The rest are not yet understood. But when we can find the cause, we usually can find a treatment." He didn't add that the treatment was correction of the deranged chemistry of the brain rather than doses of drugs that mask symptoms but do nothing for the underlying cause.

There was an old saying that some epileptics obtain their convulsions from the water faucet. This is a simplified statement concerning the permeability of the membranes of the brain cells. If it is excessive, fluid may pass which shouldn't, or in quantities which shouldn't, in either direction—into the cell or out into the brain. That explains why medical nutritionists use manganese in the treatment of some epilepsies, for this mineral helps to normalize the permeability. Traumatic epilepsies, following an injury to the brain, could be treated with octocosanol, but only a handful of physicians, even including medical nutritionists, are aware of the possibility that this natural substance, a long-chain, waxy alcohol derived from wheat germ oil, may stimulate the repair of damaged neurons—even in the brain, where such repair has always been considered impossible. Some epileptics are helped by a ketogenic diet, in which the ratio of carbohydrate to fat is so low that the body goes into ketosis, a condition that sometimes acts as an anesthetic for the nervous system.

In the Appendix, you will find the address for the Institute of Bio-Ecologic Medicine, directed by William H. Philpott, M.D. He is the physician who cared for the little girl whose history you just read. If you have a problem with epilepsy, self-treatment is obviously impossible, but your physician might be willing to query the institute for guidance to a system of natural treatment that deals with causes more than effects, and may allow you, like the little girl, to find your way to drug-free normalcy.

EYE DISEASES

- *GLAUCOMA*
- *DIABETIC RETINOPATHY*
- *MACULAR DEGENERATION*
- *EARLY POSTCAPSULAR CATARACT*
- *RETINITIS PIGMENTOSA*

Too long neglected in eye disorders, some of them ordinarily considered relentlessly progressive to blindness, are nutritional therapies, topical application of superoxide dismutase, and a ganglion-blocking technique that is advantageously used in conjunction with nutritional therapies, since it significantly increase circulation to the eyes.

In glaucoma, there are occasional patients who benefit by the diuretic effects of vitamin C (ascorbic acid) and pyridoxine (vitamin B_6). However, the basic chemistry of nutrition may be invoked to attempt reduction of elevated intraocular pressure. The medications (eyedrops) used in glaucoma are miotic drugs (causing contraction of the pupil). Biochemically, they act to inhibit cholinesterase. This is an antagonist to acetylcholine. One might describe this as approaching the problem backward, for it would be more logical to increase acetylcholine nutritionally. This can be attempted with choline, plus pantothenic acid, which is the acetylating factor, and manganese, which activates the enzyme that makes the synthesis possible. Lecithin would obviously also be helpful, as an adjunct source of choline, with the advantage that the bowel bacteria do not degrade the choline from this source, where they may attack the isolated nutrient. Information concerning these therapeutic applications of the nutrients will be supplied to physicians on request.

Now that the usefulness of vitamin E in the treatment of "neovascular disease" of the eyes in diabetics has been conceded by the *Journal of the American Medical Association,* which has long resisted the concept that this vitamin has therapeutic usefulness in human beings, more attention has been given to such antioxidants in the treatment of the visual complications of diabetes. Beneficial effects have been noted by medical nutritionists and ophthalmologists with treatment with vitamins A, C, and E, plus selenium, in retinal vascular leakage, microaneurysms, and retinal edema, with consequent improvement of sight, no more loss of sight, and no progression of the diabetic retinopathy. Occasionally, there have been reports that this nutritional therapy has improved early postcapsular cataract. Early cataract was also reported to improve, and in some cases to disappear, with topical application of superoxide dismutase in a solution of DMSO (dimethyl sulfoxide). Specifications for preparation of this solution are available to physicians only, on request. Laymen should not attempt these therapies without medical supervision, since there is a possibility of side reactions to DMSO, though I have not been able to verify any such reports. The therapeutic doses of the vitamins and the antioxidant factors—selenium and vitamins A, C, and E—will be supplied to physicians only. Supplementary amounts may, of course, be used, under the direction of the physician. These are given elsewhere for selenium (page 20) and vitamin E (page 90). Vitamin A as a supplement is used in 10,000-unit potency. Vitamin C as a supplement is used in amounts ranging from 250 mg. to 2,500 mg. daily. Therapeutic doses may be, of course, much higher.

The physician can augment the effectiveness of these nutritional therapies by performing a sphenopalatine block. This has been described by Dr. Arthur Knapp, a distinguished ophthalmologist, in numerous papers and lectures. It is performed with a tampon, moistened with Novocaine solution, which is inserted in the nose, past the second turbinate. The nerve tissue in this ganglion is quite diffuse, and accuracy in placing the tampon is not critical. The block alone has been helpful in macular degeneration and in retinitis pigmentosa, but used in conjunction with the nutritional therapies, where appropriate, it should be even more effective. The block significantly increases circulation to the eye, thereby augmenting the effectiveness of any collateral treatment. *(See also* Dry Eyes; Myopia.)

GASTROINTESTINAL DISORDERS

- *CONSTIPATION*
- *HEMORRHOIDS*
- *DIVERTICULOSIS*
- *DIVERTICULITIS*
- *APPENDICITIS*
- *BOWEL CANCER*

I have enough problems dealing with human troubles and therefore can't take time to be an expert on animal nutrition and disease, but I'd like to bet that a constipated pig is a rarity. In fact, though veterinarians may disillusion me, I shouldn't expect pigs to have appendicitis, diverticulosis, bowl cancer, or hemorrhoids. My observation is based on the fact that hogs are fed on what is removed from our flour and bread, with the result that the animal's diet shows these superiorities to white flour:

21 times the vitamin B_1	7 times the calcium
14 times the vitamin B_2	9 times the phosphorus
16 times the niacin	2 times the chromium
14 times the vitamin B_6	14 times the manganese
4 times the pantothenic acid	6 times the iron
11 times the folic acid	42 times the cobalt
17 times the vitamin E	7 times the copper
12 times the zinc	3 times the molybdenum
2 times the choline	

Those figures were compiled by Dr. Henry Schroeder of Dartmouth College, an authority on mineral metabolism, who focused his attention on the vitamins and minerals removed from our "staff of life." What he didn't comment on was what happens when we remove bran and germ from our wheat, rye, corn, buckwheat, and other starch foods; nor did he focus on the loss of fiber and nutrients in the overprocessing of sugar.

The toll for eating a diet low in fiber and nutrients that are important to digestion and elimination is extraordinarily great, but because it is so common, it is not recognized as abnormal. Constipation is a good example. We Americans buy more than 200 million dollars' worth of laxatives yearly, primarily using irritating drugs to do what good food should do: promote elimination. We suffer appendicitis—it is the most common surgical abdominal emergency in this country—and treat it as a malign stroke of the fates, rather than as a possible price for poor judgment at the dining table. We suffer with colon disorders, such as diverticulosis and diverticulitis, and with varicose veins, and yet never link these disorders to poor nutrition. Bowel cancer is so common in this country that there are colostomy clubs, formed to let old-timers, long habituated to wearing colostomy bags, induct the newcomers into the rituals of the order. This disease, too, we count as a stroke of misfortune.

The time it takes for food residues to move through the intestinal tract and exit the body is the important factor. There is a tricky point involved in defining *slow* stool transit time, for the American who is free of constipation will conclude that all is well with transit time. Actually, it is possible to have a bowl movement daily and still be the victim of slow transit. The analogy that may bring the point home is found in an automobile assembly line, where you see a completed car come off the line every five minutes and assume that all is normal, when, in fact, the car that left the assembly line a few minutes ago should have been completed last week. So it is that the bowel movement you have every day may be late. Is the point clear? The danger of delayed transit is that bacteria in the bowel have a long time in which to break down normal constituents of the stool into carcinogenic chemicals. This results in the tender tissues of the colon being bathed in carcinogens. In Central Africa, because of the high fiber content of the diet, the native is protected; his transit time is strikingly shorter. Moreover, the difference in his fiber intake and ours is only a few grams a day. The average person can appraise his resistance or susceptibility to these disorders, according to Dr. Dennis Burkitt. (He brought to our attention the remarkable freedom of Central Africans from the "civilized diseases," meaning constipation, hemorrhoids, appendicitis, diverticular disorders, varicose veins, and bowel cancer.)

Dr. Burkitt makes the observation that "the critical difference which distinguishes those who are armored from those who are vulnerable to the civilized diseases is the floaters versus the sinkers." He was saying that enough fiber in the diet to make the stool light enough to float is the protective level. The sinkers, he was saying, are the potential victims.

Eating whole wheat bread, a few slices a day, is no guarantee of adequate intake. So much is removed from our other foods, including sugar, of which we eat 125 pounds per person, per year. An enormous amount of fiber is lost to us in the processing. In addition to raising fiber intake above the critical level, it would be desirable also to try to change the intestinal flora, for the bacteria that change stool chemicals into carcinogens are distinctly not friendly; and friendly bacteria *are* available, if we change our diet.

All this led me to devise what I call the BAMBY plan. The acronym stands for:

> *B*ran
> *A*nd
> *M*ultiple vitamins and minerals
> *B*rewer's yeast
> *Y*ogurt

Other than the fiber of carrots, that from vegetables and fruits is not so effective as fiber from bran. Bran, though, isn't completely innocuous. One doesn't abruptly add a few tablespoons of bran to the diet; one doesn't abruptly stop taking it. In the early days of initial use of bran, there is a tendency to flatulence, especially if you don't increase the amount slowly. Conversely, if you abruptly cease to use bran, you will suffer constipation. Coarsely ground bran is more effective than the finely ground. You start by adding 1 teaspoon of bran to your breakfast. It's easy, if you eat a cereal or yogurt. The bran can also be incorporated in recipes for muffins, rolls, bread, pancakes, and waffles. After you have established the fact that you tolerate one teaspoonful of bran, you add another, and allow time for tolerance testing. You continue to increase until:

1. Bowel movement is effortless.
2. The stool is odorless, or virtually so. (This signals the increased transit time, which prevents the bowel bacteria from attacking the chemicals native to the stool.)
3. The stool floats, rather than sinks.

Multiple vitamins and minerals can be started as soon as the bran regime begins. A supplemental dose of vitamin B complex is also good.

Choose your yogurt carefully, for in some brands the friendly bacteria are destroyed by pasteurization. Some contain additives—gums, starch, and other thickeners, artificial flavors and colors. Those with fruits or vanilla flavoring often yield more calories from sugar than from yogurt. It is not difficult to make your own, and it is certainly less expensive. A good nutritional cookbook will explain how. You can also take lactobacillus tablets, available in the health food stores. With the friendly bacteria thereby available from two sources, you have a better chance to implant them intestinally. The claim that yogurt yields nothing but milk benefits has been refuted by a Rockefeller University paper praising the friendly bacteria of yogurt as contributing to longer life and higher resistance to infection.

There are two vitamins that are helpful. Pantothenic acid is utilized by surgeons to help patients to overcome the stasis of the intestines after anesthesia, thereby reducing the tendency to postoperative constipation and gas. The vitamin ideally would be used preventively, in supplementary amounts, before the patient is hospitalized. After surgery, the doses used medically are large. Niacinamide also benefits intestinal function, being particularly helpful in some cases of spastic colon.

Bran tablets, in 500-mg. or 1,000-mg. amounts, are available in the health food stores, as is the much less costly miller's bran. Whether the tablets are made from fine or coarse bran is relevant, but the label omits this point. One could query the manufacturer or learn by use. I usually begin with one tablet, gradually increasing the amount. To this, the fiber of carrots is a particularly useful addition. Contrary to popular concept, cooked carrots (not overcooked) are as helpful as raw.

In my experience, patients with colitis, diverticulosis, and other disorders of the intestinal tract are apprehensive about the use of bran. Experience indicates that about two-thirds of such cases are able to tolerate bran and profit by it, if initial doses are small and gradually raised.

This, incidentally, is applicable to the problem of hemorrhoids. A soft and bulky stool, eliminating the need for straining, is a sine qua non for these sufferers, and both bran and carrot fiber serve most of them well. Since a hemorrhoid is first cousin to the varicose veins that appear in the legs, it is sometimes possible to curb their development and reduce their sensitivity by the use of supplements of vitamin E (mixed tocopherol form), vitamin C, and the bioflavonoids. Doses stated on the label of the supplements would be the starting point, but, once again, your nutritionist may wish to raise these considerably. (*See also* Crohn's Disease; Ulcer.)

HEART DISEASE

Each year, for a half-million Americans, mostly male, the first symptom of heart attack is death. Cardiology, with its battery of electronic diagnostic machines, is still more an art than a science. To supplement the inadequate information yielded by the electrocardiogram

(EKG), the cardiologist turns to an "echo EKG," which bounces a signal off the heart's interior rather than recording the external electrical activity of the organ. This technique yields a little more information, but obviously not enough, and the deficit ultimately led to the technique of injecting a radio-opaque dye that would allow X-ray inspection of the heart and its vessels. But lethal heart disorders could escape that examination, too, which spurred the surgeons into developing devices to allow visual inspection of blood vessels and heart, a surgical procedure with risks, even in the most skilled hands. More information was obtained in this way, too, but *all* the diagnostic devices have a fatal flaw: The man whose heart passes the tests of the electrocardiograms isn't likely to volunteer for more drastic methods of examination, even if the mortality rate in surgical invasion of the body is "only" 1 percent—which it is in skilled hands, but that's a big 1 percent if it happens to include *you*. So it is that despite their dedicated efforts, our cardiologists have, however reluctantly, been practicing crisis rather than preventive medicine, and grasping at straws to find an effective way to reduce the deadly toll of the epidemic of heart disease.

The fact that atherosclerosis (hardening of the arteries) may start in the newborn, and may be far advanced in twenty-year-olds, as it proved to be in young soldiers who were casualties in the Korean War, emphasizes the desperate need for better screening tests. However, a new testing technique has been invented which exactly meets the needs of those whose hearts are in trouble not revealed by the older methods.

This discovery is called "nuclear cardiology." Though as yet largely unknown to both the public and some of the professions, it is a diagnostic technique that explores (and photographs) the living heart in great detail, yet without surgical invasion of the body. This is accomplished by injection of a radioactive substance into the blood. Very high-speed cameras, plus sophisticated computer enhancement of the resulting pictures, make it possible for the physician to view an actual color photograph of the beating heart, affording an accurate appraisal of heart performance, the efficiency of the pumping action, and even the stroke-volume—how much blood is ejected with each pulsation. In short, this test, which has a zero mortality rate, allows identification of the candidates for the most frequent type of heart attacks, where the first symptom of trouble is death.

Requests for the examination must come from physicians, to

whom the results are sent. To anticipate the question usually raised when radiation is involved: The amount received is approximately that which would be needed for a chest X-ray. The radioactive chemical leaves the body via the kidneys in about six hours. Thereby, the only post-test precaution is drinking generous amounts of water.

Oddly, though medical insurance carriers tend to discourage innovative medical advances by refusing payment, this procedure is covered by most policies. Unfortunately, though, in this instance the insurers are ahead of the profession, for the medical orthodoxy is putting up its usual resistance to new ideas, although the radioactive test is already in use in a number of teaching hospitals. Generally, it is the more recent medical graduates who are more receptive to the use of this technique.

That, though, still leaves you with a question of critical importance. If you take the test and it shows trouble on the horizon, what do you do? At that point, you will be the bird in a medical badminton battle. It has been said that it is the incurable disorder for which there are the most "cures." Nowhere in medicine will you find so many mutually exclusive theories as you will when you seek advice in preventing heart disease and hardening of the arteries. There are the exercise enthusiasts; the prescribers of drugs that lower blood cholesterol; those who recommend thyroid hormone treatment as prevention; the proponents of low-cholesterol, low-animal-fat diets, high in (or low in) polyunsaturated fat; those who make a panacea of high-complex-carbohydrate (starch) diets, very low in protein and all types of fat; those who emphasize the influence of heredity; those who give equal importance to stress; and those who are convinced that there is a type of personality which invites heart attacks. Central to the thesis of many of these philosophies is the belief that elevated blood cholesterol is a villain and its partner in crime is animal or saturated fat. Yet there are those who rest their case on the *type* of cholesterol in the blood rather than the quantity. Others make a persuasive case for dietary deficiencies rather than excess fat. They indict an inadequate intake of minerals and vitamins for smoothing the way for heart attacks and hardening of the arteries. Potent risk factors on which most authorities agree are hypertension (high blood pressure) and cigarette smoking. Yet, because risk factors are statistical—rather than personally inevitable—all these theories must face the reality of aged smokers free of heart disease and countries with high-fat diets (high in both animal and vegetable fat) with low incidence of heart attacks. And there are always the Winston Churchills of the world: overweight, innocent of exercise, guilty of smoking, breakfasting on brandy and a cigar, laughing at stress, and functioning in good health into advanced old age. Which is one way of saying that the only generalization that is safe is that no generalization concerning human beings is ever really safe.

So this leaves the potential heart attack victim in a quandary: What course of action to take? On what basis would you decide whether to take a drug to lower your blood cholesterol, eat one of the touted diets (some of which seem worse than heart disease), submit to a bypass operation, start jogging, discard your cigarettes, go on medication for hypertension, pop vitamin pills, or, perhaps, decide you're another Churchill. One would hope you would make your decision on the basis of reasonably valid information. But what your physician or, for that matter, the American Heart Association (A.H.A.) dispenses may not be the last word, a statement dolefully confirmed by a well-known doctor who is an ardent advocate of the A.H.A. low-cholesterol diet and an enthusiastic jogger. He wrote an article for a national magazine, titled "You Can Prevent Heart Attacks." Owing to the usual delay between acceptance and publication of an article, the doctor found himself in the hospital with his own first heart attack when the magazine reached the stands. "I am," he ruefully admitted, "disillusioned."

Let's examine the risk factors and the defenses against them. In short, let's see what precautions against heart attacks can be taken.

Stress

As a member of the board of the American Institute of Stress, I have learned a fundamental truth about stress from Dr. Paul Rosch, one of the founders of that medical society. He has presented convincing evidence that the pressures you lump under "stress" are unlikely to cause heart disease or any other stress-related disorder, provided that (1) you are good at what you do, (2) you are recognized as being good at what you do, and (3) you enjoy doing what you do. It sounds like a formula that is too pat, until you consider the enormous stress under which theatrical stars and conductors of great symphony orchestras must function, and the long, healthy lifespans many of them enjoy.

I have also learned that stress must be defined in terms of its target: The impact of the insult is determined by the soil on which it falls. Illustrative is the old jape about the husband who discovers his wife in the arms of his best friend, and comments: *"I must—but you?"* Obviously, one man's stress is another man's mistress. There is the good stress which drives us to higher accomplishment without penalty, and there is patently the bedeviling type which invites the cardiologist. Blood cholesterol is not determined by diet alone, nor by genetics alone, though that is a neglected factor; it is also modulated by stress. It rises in accountants at tax time, in medical students taking examinations, and in animals subjected to frustration. In these pressure-filled times, it may actually perform a protective function that animal experiments suggest but don't explain.

Before we leave the topic of stress, I ask you to consider a community that presents low-cholesterol and low-fat enthusiasts with the ugly fact which challenges an attractive theory. It is Roseto, Pennsylvania, a small city of second- and third-generation Italian-Americans. Their favorite dishes—like a thick slice of ham—swim in animal fat and cholesterol. Their blood cholesterol thereby is at the level Americans are warned against. Many of the citizens are overweight, including, surprisingly, the elderly, who, what with the diet and their obesity, shouldn't even be among the living. Having violated all the rules, the people of Roseto also ignore the postulated penalties. A team from the University of Oklahoma Medical School came to the small city to try to find the secret of the resistance to heart attacks, for their rate is far below the American average, and equally far below that of neighboring cities.

The answer seemed to be strong social cement. The influence of the church is pervasive and constructive. Traditions are honored. The family is a cohesive unit. Neighbors render help when needed, unasked. Young men mature with the certain knowledge of their future: They will go into the family business. But when the Roseto man moves away to *anyplace* else in America, in communities with their relative isolation and lack of social support, the demon of stress and the susceptibility to heart attacks emerges.

Lacking the social support of a Roseto, you must decide if your occupation and life-style create stresses you can't tolerate. Then you must make the decision. Will you learn how to handle stress? You *can* be taught. Will you decide if the game is worth the candle? And if it isn't, where is it written that you must play? For those who must, biofeedback is worth the trial.

Hypertension

It has long been known that high blood pressure is a strong risk factor for heart and other diseases. Before the biochemists entered the arena, the behavioral psychologists had neatly described the origin of hypertension: contention, dissension, hypertension. Today, while the emotions are still considered part of the etiology of high blood pressure, the salt-potassium ratio in the diet is regarded as more critical and perhaps more manageable. The theory starts few arguments, but the quarrel begins when treatment is considered. Orthodox therapy combines the use of hypotensive (pressure-lowering) drugs with diuretics and, frequently, tranquilizers. These medications can and frequently do cause serious side reactions. Sometimes, they actually raise blood pressure. They can cause elevated blood uric acid levels in some patients, and they all may aggravate diabetic and hypoglycemic elevation of blood insulin levels, as the price for diuretic effect. (Ironically, elevated uric acid blood levels are regarded as a risk factor for heart disease. Elevated blood insulin levels, too.) The most potent of the hypotensive drugs, used as a last resort, can cause dizziness, fainting, diarrhea, impotence—and that's only part of the list.

Of concern to the nutritionist is the loss of nutrients when diuretic medications are used to promote excretion of fluid. This effect was overlooked, as so many nutritional considerations are, in orthodox medicine, until patients began to have periods of intense weakness or fainting, traced ultimately to the loss of potassium via increased urination. Ironically, considering that hypertension is regarded as a risk factor for heart attacks, potassium deficiency is a direct threat to normal heart function. This problem was attacked in two ways: Diuretics were developed that spared potassium, and physicians began to prescribe potassium supplements. These turned out to be corrosive, serious irritation of the colon resulting from their use in some patients. As a result, the profession turned to the use of liquid potassium supplements, instead of tablets, but this didn't completely eliminate side reactions, and what should have been the first source was last tried: the foods rich in potassium, which don't cause trouble, such as orange juice, banana, tomato juice, figs, dates, raisins, and nuts. (See page 80 for a more complete list of foods high in potassium.)

This concentration on potassium losses alone was, rather than a step forward in medical thinking, another token of the blindness of the art to the importance of nutrition, for any nutritionist worthy of the title would know that other nutrients would be lost when diuretics are used. Yet to this moment, only medical nutritionists seem to be aware that diuretics cause depletion of tissue reserves in zinc. Such an induced deficiency is threatening when Americans have such limited body stores of this vital metal that one single day of fasting will be revealed by white spots on the emerging fingernails. Zinc is important in the utilization of carbohydrates, disturbances of which have been implicated in both hypertension and in types of heart disease. But then, magnesium is vital to heart function, and is probably excreted in abnormal quantities when diuretics are used. Despite this, neither zinc nor magnesium supplies are routinely replenished when these drugs are prescribed, nor have losses of other essential nutrients been explored. One must wonder what is happening to minerals other than zinc, magnesium, and potassium, and, for that matter to water-soluble vitamins, such as the B complex and vitamin C. For readers who have worshipped at the shrine of medicine and consider these apprehensions gratuitous, you might remember that disregard for life-essential nutrients caused near disaster and at least one infant death when intravenous feeding was qualitatively inadequate. My conclusion certainly doesn't smack of lese majesty: Would it not be reasonable for the physician who prescribes diuretics to protect the patient against induced deficiencies by appropriate attention to the diet and the use of multiple vitamin-mineral supplements? It is more than ironic, considering that the therapeutic effort is directed against high blood pressure, that the treatment should provoke deficiencies that may weaken blood vessels and compromise heart function.

There is no doubt that excessive intake of sodium, usually in the form of salt, contributes to hypertension in the susceptible. That term is justified, because there are those who are immune. Comparisons are available of native primitive populations, one cooking with ocean water, high in salt, the other with fresh water, the former experiencing our toll of hypertension, while the other group is not only free of it but displays a *drop* in blood pressure with aging. This is diametrically opposed to what happens in salt-soaked civilization, where for decades we were told that the "normal" blood pressure is one's age plus 100—a formula that really means that we grow sicker as we grow older. However, in this discussion we have ignored several important points. We don't know whether the craving for salt is a mark of those disposed to high blood pressure, or elevated pressure identifies those who have overindulged. We should also remember that a very large part of our excessive salt intake comes not from the salt we add, but from processed foods, and that raising potassium intake appears to be at least as important as lowering intake of sodium. (See page 78 for a list of foods and their sodium content.)

Ironically, the food processors defeat us on both points. If you look up the sodium and potassium values of a fresh vegetable, and compare them with those of a canned or frozen version of the same food, you frequently find that the potassium content has been lowered in processing and the sodium value raised.

What you have read is not the only reason for a hypertensive to avoid convenience foods. Although doctors accept as an article of faith and science that high blood pressure must be treated with low-salt diets, hypotensive drugs, diuretics, and tranquilizers, there are medical nutritionists who have scrapped this approach entirely, in favor of more natural diets, supplements, and altering of life-style. They, too, succeed in normalizing blood pressure—without the side reactions of drugs.

Even among those who pursue the traditional medical approach to hypertension, low-salt diets have been challenged because they're so difficult to follow. On a really low-salt diet, city water in some areas as well as ordinary milk and cheese couldn't be used. Milder restrictions make the diet easier to follow, but less effective. Yet many orthodox physicians consider 500 mg. of sodium daily to be an unrealistic goal, and settle for 3,000 mg. (3 g.). At any rate, salt restriction is no panacea, and as Dr. Robert C. Atkins has pointed out, both the diuretics and the salt restriction may boomerang, raising the body's output of the hormones that increase blood pressure.

Dietary calcium plays a critical role in regulating blood pressure. This is suggested not only by noting the benefits of hard water in preventing heart attacks, which I discuss later, but by many studies. A link has been found, too, between calcium deficiency and hypertension in pregnant women. Just as the ratio of sodium to potassium appears to be critical, so may the ratio between phosphorus and calcium. The American love affair with beef and other sources of nondairy protein creates a high intake of phosphorus and a low intake of calcium. With whole milk and cheese restricted in the low-cholesterol diet, and many individuals unwilling to drink nonfat milk, sources of calcium tend mainly to be the green, leafy vegetables. These are recommended by dieticians who obviously have never spent a reflective moment with the food-assay charts. What red-blooded American, in the name of preventing hypertension, would be willing to eat two to three pounds of spinach daily to confer on his macho constitution the calcium obtainable from a quart or so of milk? The result of this mindless advice is an intake of phosphorus so high that one couldn't ingest enough calcium to offset it.

This explains why the nutritionist, suggesting the use of a calcium supplement, is likely to recommend calcium orotate, if available, or calcium gluconate, rather than bone meal or dicalcium phosphate, since the last two sources serve to boost the phosphorus intake still higher.

The reliance on processed foods in our diet is another factor in high blood pressure, partially owing to the additives in these foods. Professional apologists for the processed food industry frequently assure us that *all* additives are safe. Such a blanket assurance is based on ignorance, incompetence, lies, paid association with the food industry. As an example, one of the additives included in that sweeping guarantee of safety is Red No. 3. Under another name, that dye, used in your beverages, desserts, and confections, is recommended as an insecticide for manure. It is phototoxic, photomutagenic, and photocarcinogenic, terms meaning that, if exposed to light, this "safe food additive" becomes poisonous, changes heredity, and can cause cancer.

It seems logical that since hyperactive children often improve on an additive-free diet, hypertensive adults might do likewise.

Another American habit that helps to initiate or perpetuate hypertension is our consumption of sugar, averaging a teaspoonful every thrity-five minutes, twenty-four hours per day, 365 days per year. Combined with the excessive use of caffeine, and given the stress burden the average American must tolerate, this overload of sugar disturbs the body mechanism that regulates carbohydrate metabolism. The result may be diabetes or the other side of the coin: low blood sugar (hypoglycemia). The two conditions may coexist, alternating with each other. These conditions contribute both to heart disease and to hypertension. In fact, many medical nutritionists not only will eliminate sugar intake for hypertensives but will also severely limit *all* starches and sugars during an initial period before gradually adding complex carbohydrates (starches, rather than sugars) until the optimal level is reached. Not only does this improve blood sugar levels, but such a low-carbohydrate diet is a good, natural, gentle diuretic, promoting excretion of fluid without the side reactions of drugs. For the overweight, the diet is often an effective means of reducing. (For an explanation of the characteristics that mark those who can reduce successfully only with a low-carbohydrate diet, see page 148.) *

Medicine has long recognized the value of magnesium in treating malignant hypertension. Indeed, some recent observations strengthen the evidence that lack of magnesium may be implicated in heart attacks, a reason the possible loss of magnesium from diuretics is critical. The form of magnesium best utilized by the body is magnesium orotate, which is made by combining the metal chemically with orotic acid, a normal metabolite of the body. Both vitamin C and vitamin B_6 being natural diuretics, medical nutritionists often prescribe high doses of these vitamins for their hypertensive patients. Vitamin C is used as ascorbic acid, calcium ascorbate, or magnesium ascorbate. Sodium ascorbate, a common form, would not be used, since this would be tantamount to raising the salt intake. Vitamin B_6 and magnesium enhance the action of each other, which is why taking them together is a good idea.

Since we are discussing high blood pressure as a risk factor for heart disease, it will be instructive to take a moment to watch what happens when a community shifts its water supply from soft water, which is low in magnesium and calcium, to hard water, higher in both minerals. In one Florida community, with no changes in lifestyle, a substitution of hard water for soft was followed by a striking drop in heart attacks. This relationship has been observed in cities throughout the world. Certainly, it reemphasizes the negative effect of loss of magnesium in the use of diuretic drugs, and the importance of restoring it to the diet. Illuminating, too, was the experience of a surgical team, performing open-heart surgery, who had the rare opportunity to see a heart attack start in the middle of the operation. It wasn't caused by a clot. It was a spasm, which converted soft coronary arteries into stiff, unbending vessels, hard as steel, thereby constricting circulation of blood needed by the heart muscle. In ad-

---

* It isn't relevant to the topic of hypertension, but it's worth remembering that the "optimal carbohydrate" diet, achieved by the gradual method I've described, has been a very effective treatment for depression in some patients.

dition, anyone familiar with veterinary medicine would be reminded of the tetany spasms cattle suffer in grazing on grass fertilized primarily with calcium. It is a magnesium-deficiency syndrome.

The medical nutritionist may, if necessary, tranquilize the patient with nutrients, sans the side effects of drugs. Vitamin E was described more than forty-five years ago as "dampening the transmission of anxiety impulses from the thalamus (emotional brain) to the cortex (thinking brain)." Since some elderly hypertensives react to vitamin E with rises in blood pressure, the nutritionist will give smaller than usual doses to that group and monitor the blood pressure routinely. If heart disease is present, the vitamin may have therapeutic effect; it not, the vitamin may act to prevent or mitigate heart disease. In angina, though, vitamin E might be found indispensable. I have seen angina sufferers who used 180 nitroglycerin doses monthly, and dropped to two tablets monthly after they began taking vitamin E. The vitamin can't be used with Beta-blocker drugs.

Among other calming nutrients, there is inositol, a factor of the vitamin B complex, which has a quieting effect on the brain which, displayed on an electroencephalogram, is curiously close to that of tranquilizers, *minus the side effects.* Pantothenic acid, also a B complex factor, may be used for its action in helping the body better to tolerate stress. It is also useful for the allergic person. Niacinamide, which acts upon the same cell receptors as do tranquilizers, quiets some individuals.

When vitamin C is to be administered, the nutritionist will also give bioflavonoids, factors that accompany vitamin C in foods and help its actions in the body. These strengthen the small blood vessels, an effect helpful for hypertensives, whose susceptibility to "small strokes" may thereby by reduced. The bioflavonoids also protect vitamin C from attack by oxygen in the body, which would inactivate the vitamin. They may also chelate harmful minerals, such as cadmium, which can cause or aggravate high blood pressure, thereby carrying them out of the body.

Both vitamin C and the bioflavonoids are helpful to allergic individuals. In cerebral allergy, vitamin B_6 (pyridoxine) is often given with vitamin C to reduce the symptoms. Unfortunately, hypertension specialists neglect the possible role of allergy in raising blood pressure.

The term "bioflavonoids" covers a group of substances, natural to fruits and vegetables, which are of the same chemical family. They are not, however, identical in their usefulness. Among these factors—rutin, bioflavonoids, and hesperidin—the bioflavonoids, which originate in citrus fruits, are probably the most effective, for the good reason that they dissolve more readily. Rutin is markedly insoluble, which detracts from its availability to the body.

There is a "folk" remedy for hypertension that probably works by chelating toxic minerals and dispossessing them from the body. This is garlic. For years, I thought that if garlic lowered blood pressure, it did so by keeping people away from you, but I finally realized that the deodorized product is equally effective, and so chelation of toxic minerals must be the explanation.

High- and Low-Sodium Foods and Alternatives ☐ The quantities of sodium given for the following foods are milligrams per 100 grams edible portion (about 3.5 ounces). Remember the goal: 3,000 mg. sodium daily, maximum.

3,007	Kelp	126	celery
2,400	green olives	122	eggs
1,428	dill pickles	110	cod
828	ripe olives	71	spinach
747	sauerkraut	70	lamb
700	Cheddar cheese	65	pork
265	scallops	64	chicken
229	cottage cheese	60	beef
210	lobster	60	beets
147	Swiss chard	52	sesame seeds
130	beet greens	50	watercress
130	buttermilk	45	whole milk (cow's)

Processed Foods ☐ The usual effect of food processing is to raise sodium and lower potassium content, the opposite of what we need. Be wary of the following foods because of this.

canned or frozen vegetables
smoked, cured, or canned
    meats
packaged spice mixes (not all—
    read labels)
bouillon cubes

canned fish (some are packed
without salt—read labels)
most brands of peanut butter
(have it ground fresh, in
health food store)
ketchup and barbecue sauce
potato chips and corn chips
pretzels
luncheon meats
nuts, salted
crackers, salted
soups, canned or dry
processed cheeses
salad dressings (commercial
brands)
meat tenderizers (some brands
are deliberately salt-free—
read labels.)
soy sauce
cereals with salt listed as first or
second ingredient on label

Fast Foods, High Sodium ☐ Of your allowance of 3,000 mg. of sodium daily, Burger King's Whopper and McDonald's Big Mac provide nearly one-third. Arthur Treacher's fish sandwich supplies nearly one-third; Burger King's Whaler, one-quarter; McDonald's Filet-O-Fish, 24 percent. Kentucky Fried Original Dinner gives three-quarters, their Fried Crispy Dinner, about two-thirds. A chicken TV dinner provides about two-fifths; a slice of bologna, one-fifth; ham, 13–23 percent; frankfurters, 33–42 percent; pizza with sausage and extra cheese (a 4-oz. portion), nearly one-third; canned tuna, 27 percent.

There really are no satisfactory (meaning low-salt) alternatives at the fast-food establishments, unless a fresh fish dish should be on the menu. Sliced chicken substitutes for bologna, lean roast beef will substitute for salami, and similar home-prepared meats will substitute for other delicatessen foods. Pizza is lower in sodium when no extra cheese is added. Fresh salmon substitutes for tuna. Spices, singly or in combination, rather than prepared spice mixtures, will avoid those which are heavily salted. Unsalted pretzels, potato chips, and similar snack foods are available at health food stores in some areas. Popcorn—no butter, no salt—substitutes for potato chips.

High-Potassium Foods ☐   The quantities of potassium given for the following foods are milligrams per 100 grams edible portion (about 3.5 oz.).

5,273	kelp	295	cauliflower
920	sunflower seeds	282	watercress
827	wheat germ	278	asparagus
773	almonds	268	red cabbage
763	raisins	264	lettuce
727	parsley	261	cantaloupe
715	brazil nuts	249	lentils, cooked
674	peanuts	244	tomato
648	dates	243	sweet potato
640	figs, dried	234	papaya
604	avocado	214	eggplant
603	pecans	213	green pepper
600	yams	208	beets
550	Swiss chard	202	peach
540	soybeans, cooked	200	summer squash
529	garlic	199	orange
450	spinach	191	raspberries
450	English walnut	164	cherries
430	millet	162	strawberry
416	beans, cooked	158	grapefruit juice
414	mushrooms	157	grapes
407	potato, unpeeled	146	onions
382	broccoli	144	pineapple
370	banana	141	milk, whole
370	meats	130	lemon juice
369	winter squash	129	pear
366	chicken	129	eggs
341	carrots	110	apple
341	celery	100	watermelon
322	radishes	70	brown rice, cooked

Heart Food For Breakfast

Nearly thirty-five years ago, an American physician reported the benefits of lecithin, a food substance natural to the body, in reducing the cholesterol levels in the blood, even when the diet was high in animal fat and cholesterol itself.

Despite his careful studies, those who used lecithin supplements were mocked by the antivitamin, antisupplement propagandists. Of what possible use, they asked, could it be to supplement the diet with a factor not only supplied by food, but manufactured within the body itself? Whatever impact they had, it was to the detriment of those with atherosclerosis and heart disease. Still worse, they discouraged a harmless practice that could have prevented some cases of artery and heart disease.

That becomes evident when you read a technical report, prepared in 1981 for the Food and Drug Administration by the Life Sciences Research Office, Federation of American Societies for Experimental Biology. After citing favorable effects of lecithin on memory and cognition, and in such disorders as tardive dyskinesia, Tourette's disease, Friedreich's ataxia, and disturbances caused by a drug used for Parkinson's syndrome, the report moves specifically to the cardiovascular (heart blood) effects of lecithin supplements used by mouth. The actions observed included lowering of blood plasma triglycerides and cholesterol, and actual reversal of the deposition of cholesterol in the walls of arteries.

More than twenty years before that report was issued, a chemist who was searching for relief from angina following a heart attack began to experiment with lecithin and other food factors. He didn't smoke, he wasn't overweight, he had no special stresses, he exercised liberally, and his family history was not a risk factor. In short, he shouldn't have had the heart attack in the first place. Ultimately he arrived at a simple nutritional formula in which the most active components, he felt, were lecithin and unsaturated (vegetable) oil. The recipe combines 1 tablespoon soybean lecithin in granule form, 1 tablespoon brewer's yeast, 1 tablespoon raw (untoasted) whole wheat germ (not defatted), and 1 teaspoon bone meal. The last ingredient is incorporated, says the researcher, to offset the large amount of phosphorus in lecithin. It is a choice I do not understand, since bone meal is also rich in phosphorus, and my own choice would be a calcium salt without phosphorus, such as calcium gluconate. However, I am reporting rather than improvising, and this is the formula as developed by Jacobus Rinse, Ph.D.

This mixture he made in large quantities, storing it shielded from the damaging effects of light. For breakfast, he mixes two table-spoons of the combination and adds 1 tablespoon of a vegetable oil (sunflower or safflower) and 1 tablespoon of dark brown or raw sugar for sweetening. Those who object to the sugar might use molasses. In a subsequent revision of the recipe, Dr. Rinse sub-stitute sunflower seeds for the oil, using 2 tablespoons of the seeds, on the grounds that additional and useful nutrients were provided thereby which would not be in the oil, since all vegetable oils, how-ever extracted, are overprocessed. Do not substitute other oils for those recommended since their nutritional content and amount of unsaturated molecules will vary.

The recipe is dissolved in milk, yogurt is added to improve consis-tency, and that mixture in turn is blended with cold or hot cereal, with added raisins or fruits, as desired.

For severe cases of atherosclerosis, the chemist recommended doubling the lecithin to 2 tablespoons. He also takes 500 mg. vita-min C daily, 100 I.U. of vitamin E, and a multiple vitamin-mineral supplement. The cholesterol intake from eggs and the saturated fats of butter are *not* tabooed, although he does forbid margarine. Par-tially hydrogenated fats contain an abnormal type of fat which is more of a hazard to the arteries than any of the natural animal fats. All margarines, some vegetable oils, and hundreds of American food products contain substantial amounts of these fats as a result of hydrogenation. By way of contrast, though we consume products with up to 25 percent of these fats, in Germany the ceiling is 1 percent, I am told.

The chemist, who conquered his intractable angina with this rec-ipe, points out that lecithin is like a soap. It emulsifies fats, such as cholesterol, eliminating both deposits and clots, and helps to re-move cholesterol deposits in the artery wall. His proposal, made in 1973, is now echoed by an advisory committee of the Federation of American Societies for Experimental Biology.

I have given you these data to draw upon, should the nuclear cardiology show trouble brewing in your arteries. Your physician may not be enthusiastic about Dr. Rinse's formula, and I suspect that you are likely to hear, "Well, it won't do any good, but it can't do any harm." With that license, maybe you'll teach the good doctor a lesson that will serve you and his future patients in good stead.

Chelation

I have listened to a radio interview with a surgeon rhapsodizing about triple bypass operations, which, by coincidence, he performs and about which, by equal coincidence, he has written an enthusiastic book. These are his privileges. What was not his privilege was his comment about chelation as a less risky and much less costly alternative to such heart surgery. "Oh," he said, "that's that freaky thing out of California."

I have also read statements like these about chelation:

"It's too new. We don't know enough about it."

"It's toxic to the kidneys."

"It hasn't been used on enough patients for conclusions to be valid."

Chelation is a resource that may serve you well if your arteries are hardened and circulation impeded. As honorary president of the medical society devoted to chelation,* I am in an excellent position to refute the false statements I have just quoted: Every one of them is false. It is an effective method of treating obstructed arteries without surgery; and it isn't "too new" to be judged—it's actually thirty years old. It isn't toxic to the normal kidneys, and has been used on more than 25,000 patients.

A chelating agent is one that, like a crab, extends its "claws" and grabs minerals. Chelation is a process familiar to chemists and, indeed, normal to the body. In the past, chelating agents were used primarily to sequester dangerous metals, such as lead, and convey them out of the body. Some thirty years ago, another effect of chelation was observed in one of those serendipitous events that occur with such astonishing frequency in science. A physician was treating a group of patients for lead poisoning using a chelating agent known as EDTA. In the group were several patients who had angina, and though their lead levels were the object of the treatment, it became apparent that in some unexpected way the chelation had relieved them of their heart pain.

* American Academy of Medical Preventics

This chance observation led to a trial of EDTA for the treatment of hardening of the arteries some thirty years ago. The technique involves intravenous administration of the chelating agent, which *now* requires four hours per dose, usually three times weekly for a period of some months. The term "now" is important, for in the initial experiments EDTA was administered too quickly and removed so much debris from the artery walls that the kidneys were unable to cope with their task of removing it from the body. This is where the fallacious impression was created that EDTA is poisonous to the kidneys. Experience taught the physicians that slow administration to patients with normal kidney function was as effective and much safer. Nonetheless, the illusion persisted that chelation threatens the kidneys, and that wasn't dispelled even when kidney pictures with an electron microscope refuted the allegation. As for the technique not having been used on enough patients to validate the claims made for it, I can personally report that some 18,000 chelation cases are now being placed on a computer, and that figure is but a percentage of the total.

To understand what chelation does, one must appreciate the nature of atherosclerosis. The mechanics of hardening of the arteries demand that there first be some kind of injury to the intima, the thin lining of the arteries. At the site of the injury, cells, cholesterol, and other debris from the blood will accumulate. The body attempts to interrupt the process by "plastering" this metabolic garbage, or fatty plaque, with calcium, a phenomenon that led to the mistaken belief that hardened arteries are caused by calcium. The calcification slows or halts the accumulation, but the blood vessel may be badly obstructed by the plaque; the artery itself may become brittle, and the heart ultimately affected not only by the extra work of pumping blood through narrowed vessels, but the reduced circulation that feeds the heart muscle itself.

Chelating agents can be highly selective in the metals and minerals they will eliminate, and biochemists ordinarily would not expect EDTA to pick up calcium, but it does. With the calcium sealing in the metabolic garbage, the body is powerless to remove the accumulation. Once the calcium is removed and appropriate changes in diet are made, it is possible for the condition to be reversed. Vis-à-vis this being an unproved method, you should be aware that the researchers in chelation do not rely on the patient's subjective reactions to appraise what has been accomplished in restoring circulation. Nuclear cardiography has been used to demonstrate a 54 percent increase in circulation after chelation. In addition, heat-sensitive cameras, which "take a picture" of the patient's circulation before and after chelation, show improvement after a course of treatment. These cameras, incidentally, use infrared-sensitive units of the type employed in satellites, so sensitive that from 22,000 miles away, they can detect the heat of the body of a lone swimmer in a vast stretch of ocean.

It has been recognized that chelation may remove essential nutrients other than calcium, and in the course of the treatment, these nutrients are restored. Moreover, the chelating physician does what bypass surgeons often fail to do: He prescribes necessary changes in the patient's life-style, including dietary improvement,* exercise, and cessation of smoking. If there is not sufficient improvement with an initial course of treatment, it can be repeated. In any case, the physicians who chelate suggest a refresher course of therapy at intervals determined by the patient's original condition and response to the treatment.

If the individual has normal kidney function, without which chelation is usually not administered, the only side reactions of any significance have been allergic reactions—which are extremely rare—and temporary feelings of malaise, fatigue, and lowered well-being. Called the "chelation syndrome," these reactions usually disappear in the course of the treatment or shortly following it. In some cases, the syndrome is noticed after each treatment, but patients who have had serious effects from atherosclerosis and heart disorder consider the brief reaction a small price for the benefits.

Referrals to chelation practitioners and information for physicians can be obtained from the American Academy of Medical Preventics, 8383 Wilshire Boulevard, Suite 922, Beverly Hills, CA 90211. Note that letters addressed to Los Angeles will not be delivered. The telephone number is (213) 878-1234.

Anticholesterol Drugs

Those who don't learn by experience are in deep trouble. Yet that is true of doctors—and their patients—who use drugs to alter cho-

---

* See page 82 for an example of the type of nutritional supplementing used to hold and improve the patient's response to chelation.

lesterol metabolism. The lesson that wasn't learned was taught in the trials of a medication called Mer-29. The idea behind Mer-29 was reasonable: It was recognized that the greater part of our cholesterol supply comes from the body itself, not from food. Therefore, said the pharmacologists, all that we need do is interrupt the synthesis of cholesterol in the body. Mer-29 stopped the manufacture of cholesterol at an intermediate level, but no one, apparently, had paused to wonder whether this would have adverse effects. It did. It had so many that the lawyers, pursuing suits against the manufacturer, united in a national organization to avoid duplication of effort.

Forgetting history, the pharmaceutical industry came up with another drug—clofibrate—which lowers blood cholesterol. It wasn't long before German physicians found that the drug did indeed lower the incidence of heart attacks, but at the expense of creating other diseases, with the net result that the death rate remained unchanged. The drug was banned in Germany, but American physicians still prescribe it even though they now have another equally disturbing possible side reaction to deal with. Low blood cholesterol—particularly levels below 200 milligrams percent—and susceptibility to cancer are related. But their enthusiasm for zero cholesterol was unabated. A slightly increased risk of cancer, they decided, was a price worth paying for increased resistance to heart disease, particularly when the chance of cancer is statistical, not personal. So, one might add, is the chance of heart disease. There are other side reactions, as reported by the manufacturer, in the *Physicians' Desk Reference,* where the following side reactions to clofibrate (Atromid) as listed by the manufacturer:

Cardiac arrhythmias, swelling and phlebitis at site of xanthomas, skin rash, alopecia [loss of hair], allergic reactions including urticaria [hives], dry skin and dry brittle hair, pruritis [itching], nausea, diarrhea, bloating, flatulence, abdominal distress, vomiting, stomatitis [sore tongue] and gastritis, impotence and decreased libido, renal [kidney] dysfunction as evidenced by dysuria [painful urination], hematuria [blood in urine], and proteinuria [abnormal excretion of protein], blood disturbances including leukopenia [reduction in number of white blood cells], potentiation of anticoagulant effect [tendency to hemorrhage], and anemia, myalgia [muscle aching, cramping, weakness], flu-like symptoms, arthralgia [pain in joints], fatigue, weakness, drowsiness, dizziness, headache, weight gain, polyphagia [voracious and excessive eating].

While considering what you have just read, let me add notes that strike at the fundamental thesis behind the use of such drugs as Atromid. This type of prescription writing derives from a statistical association between elevated blood cholesterol in *groups* of people and increased incidence of heart attacks. The term *"groups"* is italicized because this association is statistical, meaning that there are people with high blood cholesterol who don't have heart attacks. In fact, in one comparison of a European population with Americans of the same ancestry, the European group had a higher blood cholesterol and a lower incidence of heart attacks. And you should also know that there are many who do not accept dietary cholesterol or elevated blood cholesterol as the enemies:

1. A physician has marshaled compelling evidence that an enzyme, xanthine oxidase, which we obtain in excessive quantities from homogenized milk, can damage the artery walls and start the process of atherosclerosis.

2. A group at the Massachusetts Institutue of Technology found evidence that deficiency in vitamin B_6, quite common in the affluent nations, can cause the accumulation in the body of an intermediate substance that has the capacity to damage the artery walls. B_6 converts the toxic substance into a normal metabolite.

3. There are many thoughtful scientists who point out that we *need* cholesterol to manufacture substances vital to the body, including many hormones. In their ranks are pediatricians who protest low-fat formulas for babies. Formulas are bad enough as a substitute for breast milk, but babies *need* cholesterol to make the myelin sheaths that are the insulation for the nerves. (If you want to see what happens when these sheaths are in any way impaired, look at a person with multiple sclerosis.) Cholesterol is also vital to the brain, but the brain synthesizes its own and won't use dietary cholesterol.

4. There are biochemists who point out that cholesterol itself can't damage the artery walls; such damage, they say, must occur before a deposit of fatty plaque can start to grow. But much damage can occur from the action of highly energetic chemicals called free radi-

cals, which are formed by influences such as radiation. Normally, if our diets were adequate, they would be kept under control by the antioxidants: selenium, vitamin C, vitamin E, lecithin, and sulfur-containing amino acids. Apropos of the last, these acids are most richly supplied by eggs—which, as you know, are the first food to be forbidden in the low-cholesterol diet. Some years ago, Dr. Cuyler Hammond of the American Cancer Society reported on a study of 400,000 subjects who ate few eggs or none, compared with an equal number who ate eggs regularly. The egg-eaters, by a significant margin, outlived the egg-avoiders.

The haters of cholesterol now face a new threat to their theory. Cholesterol in the blood is wrapped in little packages, called lipoproteins, of which there are a number of types. One of these, called the low-density lipoprotein, dumps its cholesterol in the blood. Another, high-density lipoprotein (HDL), carries its cholesterol intact, dumping it where the body can excrete it. Exercise increases the level of the high-density lipoprotein, the good kind. So does alcohol (not more than two ounces daily, and none for alcoholics.) Lecithin not only reduces blood cholesterol harmlessly, but it increases HDL too. In some people, so does vitamin E.

Forgive the long explanation. I felt it was necessary if you are to accept my conclusions. First, there *are* people who can't handle saturated fats or cholesterol, but I don't tell *you* to stop eating strawberries because some people are allergic to them. Second, elevated blood cholesterol is definitely not a good idea, but an elevated level of any blood constituent is not a good idea. Third, lowering it or increasing the percentage of HDL may be wise, but there's a risk if you carry the cholesterol level below 200. Fourth, I see no reason for the risks and side reactions of drugs to control blood cholesterol levels, when there are natural ways, like the Rinse breakfast, to do that harmlessly. Fifth, I believe all the thinking about low-cholesterol diets is oversimplification of a complicated problem. Hardening of the arteries and heart attacks are certainly influenced by hypertension, cigarette smoking, lack of exercise, excess weight, diabetes, gout, inability to stand stress, excessive intake of carbohydrates (particularly sugar), and, very important, genetic differences in the ability to "handle" cholesterol. Of the last point, the Masai, in Africa, are magnificent examples. Their diet is saturated with cholesterol and animal fat, but their bodies have shut off the internal synthesis of cholesterol when the dietary supply is great.

Every fledgling scientist is taught never to use correlation to imply the cause of something. Translation: If you always see raised umbrellas when it's raining, it doesn't mean that umbrellas cause rain. Yet correlation has been repeatedly used to "prove" the case against animal fat and cholesterol as causes of artery and heart disease. Not only that, but the correlations have been hand-picked, meaning that adverse evidence, refuting the relationship, has been shouldered aside. Yet, for every country where a high-fat, high-cholesterol diet is linked with increased heart disease, you can find the opposite number somewhere: a country or an ethnic group where exactly the same diet is associated with lower levels of heart and artery disease. As for the TV commercials eulogizing vegetable oils containing no cholesterol, and actually "fighting it," you might take a close look at countries like Israel, where the cooking fat is vegetable oil and the heart attack rate as high as any in the world.

If under medical supervision you have been placed on a low-cholesterol diet and medication, and you are satisfied with your treatment and the results, what you have read obviously should not change your course. If you share my philosophy, consult with a medical nutritionist to be guided in the use of the Rinse breakfast and such supplements of vitamins, minerals, and other nutrients as tests may indicate are necessary. In either case, you will be an informed patient.

Vitamin E in the Prevention of Heart Disease

If the millions spent on drug research were only partially diverted to nutrition studies for preventing hardening of the arteries and heart disease, we might now have them under control. Lacking such funds, we have been compelled to use alternate methods of study such as those conducted by Richard Passwater, Ph.D. Dr. Passwater in a retrospective study showed that there were fewer heart attacks in those who used a vitamin E supplement; that the protection was, to an extent, proportionate to the dose; and that the protection was directly proportionate to the time span in which the supplement was used. Were that study to be repeated today, selenium would have been studied also, since its actions interlock with those of vitamin E and because deficiency in it contributes directly to heart disease, both in animals and in man. In addition to the Rinse formula, I regard it as sensible, particularly for men, but also for women approaching the menopause, to use a supplement of selenium and vitamin E. In other countries, this would not be a new idea, but the cultural lag in American medicine and particularly in American cardiology makes it so. Among veterinarians, this is old hat, for, as I pointed out earlier, they have used these supplements both for therapy and prevention for animals. Vitamin E should not be used as alpha tocopherol or any of its variations, but as *mixed* tocopherols. The potency will be measured in terms of alpha tocopherol, and from 200 to 400 units is a good supplementary intake. Selenium is best used in the organically bound form, as a concentrate derived from yeast, in a supplementary potency of 50 to 100 mcg. For those who don't tolerate yeast, which does contain a number of sensitizing substances, there is selenium from kelp, though I regard this as possibly less well utilized than the yeast form.

Vitamin B₆ (Pyridoxine) in the Prevention of Heart Disease

In the healthy body, with an adequate supply of vitamin B_6, certain biochemical occurrences result in the formation of a potentially harmful substance that, in the normal course of events, is promptly converted into a harmless and necessary final product. With a deficiency of B_6, the chain of events is interrupted at the stage where the harmful intermediate metabolite is formed, accumulates, and begins its mischief. Prolonged contact with cells damages them. A group of M.I.T. researchers believe this to be the probable cause of the initial injury to the thin lining of the artery, the lesion in which cholesterol and other debris accumulate to begin the process of hardening of the arteries. You will recall reading earlier that it is inconceivable that cholesterol itself causes the initial lesion, and that the degenerative process of atherosclerosis can't start without that "break" in the lining.

There is, however, another good reason for keeping a close eye on your vitamin B_6 intake. The vitamin is indispensable to so many processes in the body that it plays a vital role in the function of the heart muscle itself. In research never reported or expanded, a medical nutritionist back in the 1940s showed me evidence that large doses of the vitamin had reduced the size of the enlarged left ventricle, the aftermath of heart attacks in many patients. This remains unconfirmed, but protecting your vitamin B_6 intake would obviously be sensible. The vitamin is sensitive to food processing—80 percent of the pyridoxine value of wheat is lost when it is processed into white flour.

The recommended daily dietary allowance of vitamin B_6 (2 mgs. daily) is regarded by many nutritionists as much too low; they would raise it to 10 to 50 mgs. daily. As part of the vitamin B complex, it should not be used alone, but with a complete supplement of the B vitamins. Therapeutic doses of pyridoxine are higher and should be set by the medical nutritionist.

THE HYPERACTIVE CHILD

Many hyperactive children are blond and blue-eyed—deficient in pigment as compared with those of darker complexions. An amino acid—tyrosine—is used by the body to manufacture pigment, but it is also employed to create brain chemicals—catecholamines—which are the stimulating neurotransmitters. In the fair children, the theory has it that so little tyrosine is used for pigmentation that the large surplus goes to the synthesis of the brain stimulants; hence, overactivity. If the theory is correct, the hyperactivity should noticeably diminish when the children mature and, as often happens, their hair and skin darken somewhat.

However, most hyperactivity is a warning that something is wrong. And that *something* isn't a failure of your discipline, an ignorant criticism to which school systems, unable to cope with such children, subject some parents. In the largest study of its kind, over 60 percent of 200 hyperactive children given glucose tolerance tests had low blood sugar to initiate or aggravate their behavior. A large percentage of these youngsters have cerebral allergies (see page 26), which turn an everyday food—frequently one they like and eat regularly—into a trigger for behavior neither you nor the child can control. Food additives also cause problems for some children. I am aware that the American Council for Science and Health has assured the public, as has the Nutrition Foundation, that all additives are safe and don't cause hyperactivity. What they omitted from their report is the dose of additives that was tested—less than a tenth of the amount a child "normally" swallows in his daily food. When the dose was appropriately increased, some children reacted severely. Finally, some of these children are carrying a body burden of a heavy metal—lead, for example—which can subtly disturb the nervous system and the brain.

It must be more than obvious that you don't solve the problem by dosing the child with an amphetamine. Yet that is the "remedy" pediatricians prefer to an investigation of the biological disturbances I have just outlined. Amphetamines simply sedate the child, since children have a paradoxical reaction to stimulants, and you create a child whose hyperactivity is simply hiding under the facade of a sedative, his real personality never emerging.

The discussion of allergy in this text will guide you to the type of allergist who recognizes that food allergy (or maladaptive reactions to food) is a factor in many cases of hyperactivity. A medical nutritionist can conduct appropriate tests, which you can supplement by keeping an accurate food diary and a record of the child's symptoms. Links often appear: Corn flakes at breakfast was followed by destructive behavior, or the like.

Vitamin B_6 and vitamin C, used together, are sometimes successful antidotes for cerebral allergy. The medical nutritionist may wish to exceed the label doses recommended for children. The hypoglycemia diet may be needed, but there is no problem in modifying the diet for a child's needs. (See the section on hypoglycemia.) If the child shows a marked craving for sweets or an abnormal appetite for salt, this is a possible clue to the possibility of low blood sugar. The improvement in behavior when this is rectified is often startling.

Vitamin-mineral supplements, generally good protection for children, may carry some question marks for the hyperactive, since the allergic may react to vitamins, fillers, or other ingredients of the formulas. While natural vitamins and synthetic ones are equivalent, the manufacturer of natural supplements tends to avoid the use of preservatives, coal tar dyes, and the like, so that such supplements are safer. If the child has a burden of a heavy metal—say, lead—the medical nutritionist will wish to increase the intake of vitamin C and calcium to encourage excretion of the metal. In severe cases, he may wish to use a chelating agent. Vitamin C is one, but may not be adequate in treatment of high lead levels.

Don't dismiss for your child the possibility of such toxicity, low blood sugar, or cerebral allergy—not without testing.

HYPOGLYCEMIA (LOW BLOOD SUGAR)

Hypoglycemia, or low blood sugar, is not so much a disease as a symptom, and with it comes a complex of disorders of body and mind. The mental symptoms suggest need for the psychiatric couch, for tranquilizers or antidepressants, and even ECT (shock therapy); and the physical disorders range from skin diseases to arthritis, from eyesight disturbances to ulcerlike pains in the digestive tract.

When a single disorder can be the cause of so many distressing symptoms, one would anticipate that most physicians would be on the lookout for it. The opposite is true. The medical nutritionists do, but orthodox physicians have been persuaded that low blood sugar doesn't exist, that it is an "imaginary disease" invented to satisfy the need of neurotics for a physical explanation of their emotional disturbances. That is the official stance of the American Medical Association. Considering that this society has opposed virtually every advance in the science of medicine, I have come to the conclusion that if the A.M.A. opposes it, it is probably something that would benefit the public. Of this, the society itself is aware, for while denying the existence of hypoglycemia in widely circulated press releases, the A.M.A. managed quietly to offer, in its continuing medical education program, a course in the diagnosis and treatment of this "imaginary" disorder.

Otherwise competent physicians may tell you that you do not have hypoglycemia, either because it's an extremely rare condition, usually caused by a tumor of the pancreas, or because it's nonexistent. This means they are not aware that 60 percent of the patients in one large psychiatric practice were shown to have undiagnosed hypoglycemia, that the United Airlines medical department found low blood sugar in 44 or 177 pilots, that it is frequent in allergic patients, that a majority of schizophrenics have it, that some 60 percent of the hyperactive children at one treatment facility were found to be suffering from it, and that it was discovered in more than 700 of 5,000 young soldiers who had "passed" the army physical examination. Yet they persist in ignoring it; one investigator even went so far as to state that he found so many "healthy" young women to have hypoglycemia that he concluded that hypoglycemia is normal. Medical nutritionists, however, are a different story, and will do the necessary tests if they suspect the disorder. Hypoglycemia has multiple causes. The most common ones can be summed up in this acronym: SCAMS. It stands for:

Sugar
Caffeine
Allergies
Malnourishment
Stress

Even among physicians who are aware that hypoglycemia exists and know its symptoms, there are misunderstandings of the way in which a test for it should be conducted and how, when the results are at hand, they should be interpreted. It is essential that *you* understand what they do not, for hypoglycemia can wreck careers, break up marriages, lead to alcoholism, trigger asthma, or place you on a psychiatric couch when you need only to be eating a diet tailored to your needs.

We are dealing with a dynamic chemistry of the body. Sugar (glucose) levels change from minute to minute, depending on the time of your preceding meal, stress, and physical activity. When the blood sugar drops too low, or the drop is too fast, symptoms will accompany the change in those whose biochemical equilibrium is shaky. The symptoms can also appear without changes in the blood sugar level when the manufacture of insulin is too great, a point we'll discuss later.

Dr. Herman Goodman, with whom I spent years in research in hypoglycemia and other nutrition-related problems, devised a simple test that allows you, right now, to appraise the possibility that you, like millions of other Americans, have hypoglycemia. Sharpen your pencil, and follow the instructions.

Test Yourself for Hypoglycemia

Identify each symptom you have, using the four columns to rank them according to severity and frequency. 0 indicates you never have the symptom; 1 indicates that it is mild or occurs infrequently; 2 indicates that it is moderate or occurs infrequently, meaning at least once weekly; 3 indicates that the symptom is severe and frequent.

Self-test for Probability of Low Blood Sugar

0 1 2 3

_____ Tired all the time
_____ Hungry between meals or at night
_____ Depressed
_____ Insomnia
_____ Wake up after a few hours of sleep
_____ Fearful (overwhelmed by people, places, or things)
_____ Can't decide easily
_____ Can't concentrate
_____ Poor memory
_____ Worry frequently
_____ Feel insecure or low self-image
_____ Highly emotional
_____ Moody
_____ Cry easily or feel like crying inside
_____ Fits of anger
_____ Magnify insignificant details (create mountains out of mole hills)
_____ Eat candy or cookies, drink soda pop
_____ Eat bread, pasta, potatoes, rice or beans
_____ Consume alcohol
_____ Drink more than 3 cups of coffee or cola drinks daily
_____ Crave candy, soda, or coffee between meals or midafternoon
_____ Can't work well under pressure
_____ Headaches
_____ Sleepy during the day
_____ Sleepy or drowsy after meals
_____ Lack of energy
_____ Reduced initiative
_____ Eat when nervous
_____ Stomach cramps or "nervous stomach"
_____ Allergies: asthma, hay fever, skin rash, sinus trouble, etc.
_____ Fatigue relieved by eating
_____ Suicidal thoughts or tendencies, feelings of hopelessness
_____ Bored
_____ Bad dreams

HYPOGLYCEMIA (LOW BLOOD SUGAR)

0 1 2 3

_____ Irritable before meals
_____ Heart beats fast (palpitations)
_____ Get shaky inside if hungry
_____ Feel faint if meal is delayed
_____ Ulcers, gastritis, chronic indigestions, abdominal bloating
_____ Cold hands or feet
_____ Trembling (shaking) of hands
_____ Blurred vision
_____ Bleeding gums
_____ Dizziness, giddiness, or light-headedness
_____ Aware of breathing heavily
_____ Bruise easily
_____ Reduced sex drive
_____ Uncoordination (drops or bumps into things)
_____ Sweating excessively
_____ Unsocial or anti-social behavior
_____ Muscle twitching or cramps
_____ Skin aches
_____ Phobias
_____ Hallucinations
_____ Convulsions
_____ TOTAL

Add the total number of symptoms checked in each column—1, 2, and 3—and multiply the number of checks in each column by the number at the top. Now add the three totals.

If your score is under 20, there is but 1 chance in 20 that you have low blood sugar.

If the total score is 20–25, the possibility of a glucose tolerance test showing abnormality is about 50 percent.

If the total score is between 35 and 45, the chance of an abnormal glucose tolerance test rises to 90 percent.

A score over 45 indicates that there are only 2 chances in 100 that your glucose tolerance test will be normal.

Remember that this test is a rough measure of probability—not a diagnosis. If your score indicates the possibility of disturbed sugar metabolism, you should consult a qualified physician and discuss your having a glucose tolerance test or, if he elects, therapeutic diagnosis. This, you will recall, is obtained by watching your response to the hypoglycemia diet, improvement usually meaning that you needed the diet because you did in fact have hypoglycemia.

Translating the results of the test into action is imperative if your score falls into the danger zones. That means going to a competent physician for appropriate medical and nutritional testing, rather than learning the lesson the hard way, as did a reader who wrote: "Tell your readers not to be stupid as I was. I scored over 45 on your home test for possible hypoglycemia, but I ignored that and went on suffering with all those symptoms for another six months before I finally went to a physician and had the glucose tolerance test for hypoglycemia. The test was positive; in fact, I had such severe symptoms during the second hour that they stopped the test. I was put on the low blood sugar diet, and I feel fine, for the first time in years."

Going to a competent physician isn't a stock phrase. In the tens of thousands of letters I've received from readers of my book on hypoglycemia, there is one from a college professor who had to fight with his physician to receive a glucose tolerance test, and though during the test he went into convulsions, lost his color vision, and stammered incoherently—all this from a dose of sugar!—the test results were called "normal." This happened at a major hospital associated with a major medical school. To further justify my caution in selecting physicians for hypoglycemia, let me show you how 1,100 hypoglycemics were misdiagnosed on the basis of their symptoms. They were studied by a physician who himself had the disorder. The following symptoms appeared in 50 percent or more of the patients: nervousness, irritability, exhaustion, faintness, dizziness, tremor, cold sweats, weak spells, depression (77 percent of the patients), vertigo, dizziness, drowsiness, headaches, digestive disturbances, forgetfulness, constant worrying, unprovoked anxieties, insomnia of the type where the patient awakens in the small hours and is unable to return to sleep, a feeling of internal trembling, mental confusion, palpitation of the heart, rapid pulse, muscle pains, numbness, and indecisiveness.

In more than 27 percent of the patients, there were these added symptoms: unprovoked weeping, lack of sex drive (particularly in females), allergies, uncoordination, leg cramps, lack of concentration, blurred vision, twitching and jerking of muscles, itching and crawling sensations on skin, gasping for breath, smothering spells, staggering, sighing and yawning, impotence, and night terrors and nightmares.

More than 17 percent of the patients had these added symptoms: unconsciousness, rheumatoid arthritis, unjustified fears, neurodermatitis, suicidal intent, and symptoms interpreted as "nervous breakdown."

Two percent of the patients had the most violent symptom of all: convulsions. These patients were never diagnosed as having hypoglycemia. This is a list of what they were told they were victims of: mental retardation, neurosis, "slight nervousness," hives, neurodermatitis, Ménière's syndrome (loss of hearing, dizziness, and noises in the ears), atherosclerosis of the brain, pain in the head, asthma, rheumatoid arthritis, Parkinson's syndrome ("senile palsy"), rapid beating of the heart (tachycardia), "imaginary sickness," menopause, alcoholism, and diabetes. Several were told they had overproduction of insulin, the correct diagnosis, but were told to eat candy—which makes it worse!

The Glucose Tolerance Test

The glucose tolerance test is relatively simple a medical procedure, and one would think it virtually foolproof. The patient's fasting blood-sugar level is determined; he is given a dose of sugar (glucose), usually 100 g., which is about 3⅓ ounces; and then his blood sugar levels are monitored at regular intervals—usually every half-hour for the first hour and then every hour to six hours. This is in sharp contrast to the quick test for blood sugar—pricking the finger and determining the blood sugar level at the moment. This may reveal an elevated level suggesting diabetes, but it tells nothing about the dynamics of sugar metabolism hour by hour.

There are many objections to the standard glucose tolerance test, and some of them are troubling. The test is usually conducted in the peace and quiet of the laboratory or the doctor's office, and the results may be far removed from what happens to blood sugar levels when the patient is exposed to the stresses of everyday activities. Then, too, allergy is characteristic of hypoglycemics, and corn allergy is a frequent one, which is pertinent because glucose is made from corn. This raises the (usually) unanswered question: Is the patient reacting to the sugar, its source, or both? The use of glucose itself is open to challenge. Most hypoglycemics are saturated with sugar, which is not solely glucose, but a 50–50 combination of fructose (fruit sugar) and glucose. Should not sugar be used in the test rather than glucose? In many medical offices, the glucose solution is cola-flavored. This is more than a mistake; it is stupid, for most cola contains caffeine, to which hypoglycemics react adversely, and which may distort the test results, for caffeine, by stimulating the adrenal glands, induces the liver to discharge sugar into the blood.

To compensate for the lack of stress in the laboratory setting, some physicians will, at the fourth hour of the test, have the patient run on a treadmill or pedal a stationary bicycle, or hyperventilate by breathing rapidly into a paper bag. Frequently, this will have a demonstrable effect on the following test of blood glucose level.

Other physicians, mostly medical nutritionists, aware of the deceptiveness of the peace-and-quiet environment for blood sugar determinations, have the patient report before breakfast, to determine the fasting sugar level; after breakfast, to appraise what his morning meal does to it; and then at intervals during the morning, before and after lunch, up to midafternoon. This certainly gives a more accurate picture of the patient's carbohydrate metabolism during normal activities, and it may differ sharply from the results of the tests in the laboratory environment. The method has one disadvantage: The physician can't observe the symptoms of the patient, to correlate them with the blood sugar levels. He must rely on the patient's own reports, and many doctors distrust subjective observations. On the other hand, some doctors pay no attention to symptoms evoked by blood glucose changes, as indicated in the story about the college professor. This difficulty is created by what I call the "magic number" school of thought, which says that you don't have low blood sugar unless the level drops below a certain number. The fact is that people's metabolisms have no respect for standard numbers, and I have *seen* patients undergoing a glucose tolerance test who went into convulsions with the blood sugar well above the "magic number." This is the obvious reason for a warning: Never submit to a glucose tolerance test if you are left alone in the laboratory or the physician's office. The magic number philosophy completely disregards the patient's reactions to the test, which are just as much an index of disturbed carbohydrate tolerance as the test numbers. If vision is blurring, speech becomes thick, thinking becomes clouded, unprovoked crying occurs, or convulsions result (which happens in a small percentage of patients), it doesn't matter what happened to the glucose blood level. Whatever it is, the patient obviously can't tolerate it, and the doctor must remember that suspicion of such intolerance is the motivation for the patient's visit, in many cases.

The magic number myth also disregards completely the possibility that normal blood glucose levels are accompanied by excessive high blood insulin levels. Elevated insulin activity can create all the mischief usually associated with low blood sugar. In fact, it is my prophecy that glucose tolerance tests without measuring blood insulin levels will one day be regarded as a disservice to the patient.

There are several tests for hypoglycemia, other than the six-hour glucose tolerance. One is a screening test that Goodman and I developed some ten years ago. It requires but an hour: If within that period, in response to the usual dose of glucose, the blood level does not rise at least 50 percent, the six-hour test will probably reveal hypoglycemia. If it rises more than 100 percent, the six-hour test will probably show diabetes. Another test, developed by Dr. Carl C. Pfeiffer at the Brain Bio Center in Princeton, New Jersey, measures other blood chemicals, spermine and spermidine. These are related to histamine, and the test also correlates well with hypoglycemia. Hair tests are useful only when interpreted in the light of other findings, such as blood and urine chemistries. I mention this because the public has been persuaded that hair tests for minerals are a complete answer to diagnostic problems involving these minerals. Not so, and a good example is the elevated sodium frequently found in the hypoglycemic's hair. The layman or the inexperienced physician will interpret this to indicate that the body has an excess of sodium, when the fact is that this represents excess *excretion,* which is creating salt *deficiency* and which points to the possibility that the adrenals, which help us to retain salt, are not functioning normally. Do not submit to hair analysis unless expert interpretation, fortified by results of complete physical and biochemical examinations, is available.

Hyperinsulinism versus Hypoglycemia

Earlier, I promised to explain the relationship of blood insulin levels to symptoms of hypoglycemia in patients who definitely *don't* have low blood sugar. They are often cited to "prove" that low blood sugar is imaginary, but they actually demonstrate that elevated *blood insulin levels* can cause every symptom of hypoglycemia, though blood sugar deficits or rapid drops are not present.

Excessive concentrations of insulin can cause every disturbance, every symptom that has ever been reported in hypoglycemics. The high-insulin patients with normal blood sugar tend to fall into three groups:

1.   The elevated insulin levels cause gastrointestinal symptoms such as cramps, diarrhea, or the ulcerlike pains frequently present in low blood sugar.

2.   Elevated insulin levels can cause the "emotional" and "mental" symptoms characteristic of many hypoglycemics.

3.   When in response to a dose of sugar, the insulin levels rise, but the rise is delayed, this may be a warning of latent diabetes.

I am puzzled by one aspect of this type of hyperinsulinism: Why don't the elevated blood insulin levels cause hypoglycemia in this group of sufferers? You may be puzzled by another: Why does elevated blood insulin cause the symptoms of low blood sugar? It appears to be little realized that excessive amounts of insulin can gravely disturb the permeability of the cell membranes in the brain. Such an action can create chaos in brain chemistry and trigger adverse effects on the nervous system.

When you realize that the treatment for hypoglycemia and for elevated blood insulin levels is the same—a low-sugar diet—all this may seem an academic tempest in an oversweetened teapot. In a sense, yes, but you must remember that the person with elevated blood insulin levels whose test for hypoglycemia is negative will be told that his disease is imaginary and that he needs a shrink and a tranquilizer, not necessarily in that order.

Therapeutic Diagnosis

To me, after forty years of study of hypoglycemia, both in theory and in clinical observation, the best method of testing for the condition is therapeutic diagnosis. That translates as bypassing the test, placing the patient on the hypoglycemia diet, and observing his reactions. If the symptoms disappear, the diagnosis is confirmed. Philosophically, medicine should have no reservations about therapeutic diagnosis. It is used (and approved) when colchicine is given to treat a painful big toe when the diagnosis of gout is in question. Since the drug is effective only against gout, the disappearance of pain and swelling in response to it make the diagnosis.

What if therapeutic diagnosis is used and fails? That happens, though it is rare in patients who score high on the self-test for hypoglycemia. The patient has gained by better nutrition, which the hypoglycemia diet represents, and the glucose tolerance test can always be given. If that test is positive, despite the fact that the patient has not responded to the diet, there are five possibilities:

1. The patient is allergic to foods in the diet, and those allergens must be removed from it.

2. The amount of carbohydrate allowed in the usual high-protein hypoglycemia diet is not enough or too much for this particular patient. As little as 20 or 30 g. of carbohydrate—up or down—can make the difference.

3. The patient is under too much stress. The term "stress" does not always, in this context, mean chaotic pressures. There is also the stress of a life-style that offers no sense of accomplishment, no pride, and no rewards. This tends to produce what the physician calls the "flat glucose tolerance curve." It is often associated with allergy, too.

4. The adrenal glands need support.

5. The patient (always a woman, in this instance) has the rare Morgagni's syndrome, which presents all the symptoms of hypoglycemia, with a normal glucose tolerance test, and does not respond to the usual hypoglycemia diet unless it is supplemented with a source of glycine (whole gelatin).

We must return to reasons 3 and 4 for failure of the diet to relieve the symptoms. Though they do not appear to overlap, they actually involve the same mechanism: adrenal failure. Where the patient's life-style is monotonous, filled with tedium, and devoid of a sense of accomplishment, the flat curve results, where blood sugar does not rise normally in response to a dose of sugar, and instead of peaking and then falling, which is the normal curve, stays at an inadequate level virtually throughout the test. Allergy can be behind this, but so can psychosomatic forces—that is, the adrenals are not responding by raising blood sugar because there is no challenge in the life-style. Adrenal function can also be directly disturbed, meaning that these glands in the hypoglycemic must fight a running battle with the pancreas, with insulin lowering the blood sugar, and adrenal hormones produced in an effort to raise the level to normal. This mechanism is so delicate that one authority has said that a drop of blood sugar of only 3 mg. (normal fasting level is between 60 mg. and 100 mg., we are told) forces the adrenal glands into compensatory activity. In most hypoglycemics, the adrenal failure is relative to the overactivity of the pancreas, and once that organ has been quieted by a low-sugar diet, the adrenals return to normal. In some, the glands become directly exhausted and remain so even after the pancreas has reduced its insulin output to normal.

The physician has resources to appraise the adrenals. Weak adrenal glands cause hypoglycemics to "dump" salt. They also permit excessive salt accumulation in the hair, detectable by a hair analysis. If these tests indicate that the adrenals need rest and recovery, the physician can prescribe vitamin C, PABA, and pantothenic acid to stimulate the gland, give glandular therapy (dried adrenal tissues) by mouth, or, which was customary until the FDA stupidly interfered, inject adrenal cortex. The FDA, cooperating with the A.M.A. in an effort to discourage medical interest in hypoglycemia, declared that adrenal-cortex-injectable products do not have enough cortisone to be useful. The cortisone content is of no interest to the medical nutritionist, but the many other hormones in the cortex are—and they are helpful to hypoglycemics. Efforts are under way to dissuade the FDA from interfering with the practice of nutritional medicine. The relationship between the competent physician and his cooperative and informed patient is too close to allow the intrusion of a government agency which, after all, has never been licensed to practice medicine or to regulate how it should be practiced. The adrenal cortex extract (known to physicians as ACE) is helpful for all hypoglycemics whose adrenals do not recover fully with the hypoglycemia diet and, very practically, for those who initially benefit by the diet and then strike a plateau with incomplete recovery, and are left with residual symptoms, the most frequent of which are impotence in the male and frigidity in the female. Such residual symptoms are particularly frequent in patients with the "flat curve." When the flat curve is the externalization of tedium and an unchallenging life-style, neither the diet nor adrenal cortex injections will effect a total or lasting benefit. This is the one type of hypoglycemia where psychological support, and, indeed, psychotherapy in aggravated cases, will become indispensable. This is to say that the "tired housewife syndrome" often is the symptom pointing to hypoglycemia and a flat glucose tolerance curve, but permanent help will not come from diet, vitamin supplements, and adrenal cortex injections until the tired housewife is persuaded that she is a valuable and needed member of the family and community.

The Hypoglycemia Diet

There are some dietary principles that are applicable to all hypoglycemics. The timing of meals is as important as their content. Six small meals daily, or three larger meals plus three snacks, are mandatory. The three-meal-per-day pattern of eating has nothing to do with physiological needs. It is a concession to our bus schedules, business duties, household obligations. Rather than going from fasting to plenty and back to starvation level again, three times daily, hypoglycemics profit by minimizing these changes.

Each of the meals and snacks should contain a small portion of protein—as little as an ounce—in the smaller feedings. This has behind it a scientific truth which is recognized in the old phrase, "A steak sticks to your ribs. Bread leaves you hungry an hour later."

Both the amount of protein and the amount of carbohydrate ideal for the individual *are* individual. We usually start with 60 gm. of complex carbohydrate, starch rather than sugar, daily, and half your body weight in grams of protein. This would mean 55 gm. protein for a 110-pound woman, for example, taken from meat, fish, fowl, cheese, eggs, milk, yogurt, and other high-quality protein sources. The 60 gm. of starches—bread, potato, whole grain cereals, etc—is a starting point. I have seen hypoglycemics who recovered beautifully at the 60-gm. level. I have also seen those who remained tired until we doubled that. Sometimes, even a half of a baked potato, twice a day, is the critical addition needed. In this endeavor to regain your health, you must not ask the physician to solve all the problems. It requires that you take charge of your own body.

There are those who claim to have all the answers, to have one type of diet that is the panacea, not only for low blood sugar but for virtually all other diseases. Particular offenders are those who label high-protein diets a "big mistake" and urge sole use of a high-carbohydrate, low-protein, and low-fat diet—the same approach they use for heart disorders and atherosclerosis, with equally inflated claims. Yet the diet that precedes the onset of hypoglycemia in the large majority of patients is not high-protein. They didn't arrive at low blood sugar by eating eggs for breakfast; they chose Danish pastry, or doughnuts, or toast and coffee. Their lunches weren't high-protein; more often than not, they lunched on sandwiches with a skimpy protein filling, offering more calories from starch (bread) than from protein. With luck their evening meal was adequate in protein, but conveyed another dollop of starch and sugared desserts. Their snacks between meals *were* carbohydrates—from potato chips to pretzels—and their beverages were sugar-saturated soda pop. One does not repair liver dysfunction solely by eating a high complex-carbohydrate diet. Protein is needed. Optimal carbohydrate intake must be established for every hypoglycemic individually. (Indeed, we'd all be better for arriving at it.)

The technique for establishing optimal carbohydrate intake is described in the discussion of depression on page 43.

Most hypoglycemics picture the low-carbohydrate diet as a kind of penance for their dietary sins. A sample menu for one day demonstrates that it requires only a little thought and effort to arrive at an adequate (or therapeutic) diet for a hypoglycemic, without taking the pleasure away from eating.

Sample Menu with Recipes

BREAKFAST

6 oz. tomato juice
Eggs in Nests
½ slice toast, whole wheat or whole rye, with 1 tsp. butter
coffee (decaffeinated), weak tea, or herb tea (no sugar).

Eggs in Nests: For two, use 4 eggs, 2 tbsp. nonfat dry milk, ¼ tsp. tarragon, and salt and pepper to taste. Separate whites and whole yolks. Beat whites to stiffness, add powdered milk and seasoning, and rebeat until peaks form. Pile whites into Pyrex cup. Make depressions in middle for yolk. Place yolks in depressions, top with a little tarragon, and bake until yolks set and whites turn golden brown—usually 20 minutes at 375° F. Two yolks for you. Where high protein does well by you, a teaspoonful of cottage cheese can be added to each depression before yolks are inserted.

MORNING SNACK

1 cup skim milk with ¼ cup creamed cottage cheese

When you tire of plain skim milk, add a little vanilla, papaya juice, or carob powder. Carob tastes like chocolate but doesn't stir up chocolate allergies or create acne problems, as chocolate sometimes does. It is available in health food stores, and contains some carbohydrate, which must be deducted from the 60-gram intake, unless you have discovered you need more carbohydrate.

When plain cottage cheese palls upon you, add horseradish, caraway seeds, poppy seeds, shredded spinach, chopped chives, chopped onion or scallion, chopped dill, etc.

LUNCH

Crab salad in gelatin on tossed green salad
sliced fresh tomato with vinegar and vegetable oil dressing (Do not use oils that contain BHA or BHT as preservatives. Read labels.)
Tea South of the Border

Crab salad: Dissolve 1 tbsp. unflavored whole gelatin in ¼ cup cold water. Add 1 cup plain chicken consommé, 3 tbsp. white wine or lemon juice, dash of Tabasco if desired. Stir and chill, and just before it becomes thick, add 1 cup cooked flaked crab meat, either fresh or canned, ½ cup diced cucumber, ¼ cup chopped celery, ¼ cup chopped green pepper, and ¼ cup thin-sliced radishes. Chill in mold for several hours and serve on green salad, flanked by tomatoes.

Tea South of the Border: Brew tea, not too strong. Boil three cinnamon sticks in quart of water, and add brew to tea in quantity that pleases you. If you want sweetening, use saccharin.*

AFTERNOON SNACK

½ cup skim milk
Tongue Horn

Tongue Horn: Press pot cheese through strainer. Add just enough yogurt to work it to a soft paste. Add chopped dill or chopped dill pickle. Roll ¾ oz. of this in very thin tongue, leftover roast beef, or ham.† Secure with toothpick to make small horn.

SUPPER

⅛ cantaloupe, with dash lime or lemon juice
Liver á la Fredericks—3 oz. for you
Bibb lettuce, 2 tsp. mayonnaise (avoid brands with partially hydrogenated fats)
thin carrots
pears in ginger jelly
decaffeinated coffee, weak tea, or herb tea

Liver à la Fredericks: Use beef, pork, or lamb liver—your choice. Render some butter. Add seasoning to taste. Brown a chopped onion. Bread liver—no bread crumbs—using a little wheat germ, and slice into strips about the size of macaroni. (Your butcher can do this better, unless you have a very sharp knife.) Add breaded liver strips to onion and butter mixture as browning begins. Cook only a

---

* Knowing from experience that the mention of saccharin will bring anxious inquiries about the reputed dangers of the artificial sweetener, let me note first that you must not abuse it as, possibly, you have abused sugar. Second, the United States banned cyclamates on the grounds of possible bladder cancer, while Canada banned saccharin on the same grounds, and the bladder cancer rate in the two countries is the same. I do not believe that a small amount of the sweetener poses a threat.

† There is a very real risk in eating meats containing nitrites or nitrates. The risk can be largely eliminated if vitamin C and vitamin E are taken immediately after the meal.

few minutes, all told, on both sides, and quickly. Overcooked protein isn't as good for you.

Thin carrots: Melt butter with seasoning to taste. Add wafer-thin carrot slices. Cook only until yellow color begins to run into butter. Top, if desired, with a little tarragon.

Pears in ginger jelly: Sprinkle 1 envelope unflavored whole gelatin into ¼ cup cold water and let stand for 5 minutes. Then place in double boiler and stir until gelatin is completely dissolved. Remove from heat, add ¼ cup ginger brandy and 1½ cups artificially sweetened ginger ale, and blend. Canned pears (water or self-juice pack) should be drained and sliced; fresh, peeled and sliced. Sprinkle six pears with a little ginger brandy and chill. At serving time, arrange the sliced pears in a glass bowl, topped with the jelly. One pear is the normal portion; yours is one-half pear.

NIGHT SNACK

Ground Meat Pizza
Add a pinch of pepper to I lb. lean ground beef and knead. Line 6-inch Pyrex dish with meat as substitute for ordinary pizza pastry shell. Chop 4 fresh tomatoes, mix with 2 tsp. diced onions to make paste, add ¼ tsp. each of oregano, paprika, and sweet basil. Fill meat shell with this mixture, lightly season with oregano on top and bake at 350° F. to doneness you prefer. Your snack is 1 oz.; let the family enjoy as much as they want.

If however, like many hypoglycemics, you don't feel like fussing with the type of gourmet low-carbohydrate menu you've just read, you can choose the simple menu. Here is one that is spartan and easy to prepare.

BREAKFAST

½ grapefruit
1 poached egg
1 oz. chicken or leftover meat
½ slice whole wheat toast
1 tsp. butter

MORNING SNACK

1 cup skimmed milk
¼ cup creamed cottage cheese

LUNCH

Chicken or tuna salad with 3 oz. (about ¾ cup) tuna or chicken
4 tsp. mayonnaise (without partially hydrogenated fats)
chopped celery
green beans with 1 tsp. butter
sliced tomato
beverage

AFTERNOON SNACK

½ cup skimmed milk
1 oz. American or Cheddar cheese

SUPPER

3 oz. steak
cauliflower with 1 tsp. butter
tossed salad with vinegar and oil dressing
2 halves canned peaches (water or self-juice pack)

EVENING SNACK

½ cup skimmed milk
1 oz. pot cheese, softened with a little yogurt and wrapped in thin slice beef

Note: If, with your hypoglycemia, you are also overweight, it is important that your vegetable oil intake be precisely measured. You need 5 tsp. daily to accelerate weight loss. It will be slow without it, and you must not exceed the 5 tsp.

Supplements in Hypoglycemia

The allergies of many hypoglycemics will interfere with or force modification of the program of supplementing, for the allergic will manage sometimes to react adversely to vitamins they need or to the fillers, excipients, colors, and preservatives in many vitamin products. While natural and synthetic vitamins are equivalent, I prefer vitamins of natural origin for hypoglycemics (and, not incidentally, for all children) for the reason that manufacturers of the natural products tend to avoid the use of fillers and additives. Most hypoglycemics profit by a multiple vitamin-mineral supplement, plus a vitamin B complex concentrate. If tolerated, a natural source of the vitamin B complex is added to arrive at a supply of the "unknown" factors, known to be present, known to be useful, but not available isolated. Desiccated liver is the first choice. If it's not tolerated, use brewer's yeast. Since both these foods are highly allergenic, we are sometimes forced to go to useful but less desirable sources of the natural B complex, such as wheat germ (not defatted, and always vacuum-packed, if obtainable) and rice polishings.

Liver function is part of the problem of hypoglycemia, though excessive attention has been directed to the pancreas. For this reason, the B-complex concentrate should provide 1,000 mg. choline and 500 mg. inositol in the recommended daily dose. If such a formulation is not available, one can use any B-complex supplement and purchase the inositol and choline separately. Some manufacturers combine them in one tablet; some add methionine, an amino acid that is also helpful to liver function. Lecithin, particularly the high-phosphatidyl choline type, is useful for hypoglycemics, particularly those troubled with anxiety and those whose tolerance for fats is limited. The physician may prescribe high doses of all these concentrates. The supplementary doses are those stated on the labels.

A hypoglycemic's cocktail has been invaluable to many sufferers. It has a triple purpose:

1. It is a prebreakfast drink to build energy reserves for the day, taken before rising.

2. It is a prebedtime drink, to help minimize the small-hours drop in blood sugar that is innocuous to normal people but may be aggravated in hypoglycemics, causing them to awaken and have difficulty in returning to sleep.

3.   It is also used when awakening does occur, to help return to sleep.

The recipe is pretty much to taste, but a typical one starts with nonfat milk powder. The quantity normally used to make a quart is used to prepare a pint, or at most, a pint and a half, dissolved in water. This is blended with the yolks of two eggs, a teaspoonful of vanilla (optional), and three tablespoonfuls of U.S.P. glycerin. The glycerin is used for two purposes: It is sweet enough to satisfy those who still crave that quality, and, more important, glycerin is converted into "stored sugar" (glycogen) in the body. This does not raise blood sugar, but can be drawn on for that purpose when the body needs the fortification. A glassful is taken before arising, before bedtime, or as needed if awakening does occur. When for some reason breakfast must be skipped, despite the importance of a good one for hypoglycemics, a glassful of the "cocktail" is a good if makeshift substitute. It must be remembered, though, that milk does contain sugar (lactose), and the amount in a quart of milk, whether nonfat or whole, is nearly an ounce, some 28 g. This must be counted as part of the total carbohydrate intake for the day.

Supplementary *rest* is also sometimes medicinal for hypoglycemics. Those who find it difficult to get started in the morning will often find it helpful to rise, have breakfast, and return to bed for an hour. If earlier rising is necessary to do this, the investment is worthwhile, for the practice seems to make more efficient the "recharging" of the hypoglycemic's "batteries."

If you have reason to suspect that you are a victim of hypoglycemia or its twin, elevated insulin levels, don't allow anyone—with whatever professional degree or other cloak of authority—to interfere with your obtaining competent diagnosis and treatment. Low blood sugar can make *any* disease worse. It may incite or worsen asthma. It can masquerade as neurosis, imitate psychosis, stimulate schizophrenia or worsen it, incite alcoholism or perpetuate it, initiate or intensify allergy, imitate arthritis or increase its aches and pains, put multiple sclerosis patients in wheelchairs, create or intensify reading and learning difficulties, aggravate hyperactivity, cancel the sex drive, initiate suicidal depression, and perfectly imitate or worsen epilepsy—and that is only a partial list. Syphilis was once called "the great masquerader," but hypoglycemia deserves that title.

INFERTILITY

Infertility is the problem of one couple in every ten. This may come as a shock if you've been impressed by all the baby carriages you see and the endless television advertisements for paper diapers, but the fact is that the reproductive inefficiency of modern man and woman would not be tolerated in stables where they raise thoroughbred horses that have a high cash value.

Reproductive efficiency is one of the basic criteria for evaluating the worth of a diet, for it must allow you to enter the world, help you to mature, maintain your health, and permit you to reproduce. Measured by those standards, the American diet is in trouble, and we are, too. Consider modern food, with its additives, pesticides, residues, and the overprocessing to which it has been subjected; it isn't particularly astonishing that it is a weak link in supporting reproduction. Yet it is the last consideration, if, indeed, it is considered at all, in solving the problem of an infertile couple. I find this paradoxical, not only because nutrition is a veterinarian's important weapon in helping reproduction in valuable animals, but because there are literally hundreds of babies for whom I am nutritional godfather, born to families who had been infertile until they were persuaded to change their diets.

"Their diets" means the menus for both the would-be father and mother. This goes far beyond the mere counting of sperm and appraisal of sperm motility, which are the usual standards by which male fertility is measured. It certainly goes beyond allowing a malnourished woman to become pregnant, to eat even more inadequately through early weeks of morning sickness, and then to place herself on a self-selected diet of "typical American foods." Not that this projection is the most dismal one could make. There is another alternative: The expectant mother falls into the hands of an obstetrician who prescribes a low-calorie, low-protein, low-salt diet, accompanied by diuretics. He is trying to prevent pregnancy toxemia or pregnancy eclampsia. The surest cause of those conditions is the malnutrition his regimen will produce. It is SPUN (The Society for the Protection of the Unborn Thru Nutrition), of which I am a member, which named it: "thalidomide #2."

Returning to the problems of the infertile couple, I would place both partners on a good diet for at least six months before conception is attempted. (It's not so radical as it sounds. In the South Seas, I am told, there are primitive groups who will not permit a couple to attempt conception unless they have both been on a special diet for a significant period of time.) I should wish to supplement that diet, because overcoming years of indifferent nutrition requires more potent intake of vitamins and minerals than food alone can supply.

None of this, of course, replaces a complete physical examination and necessary corrective measures for both partners. What I am not including in "corrective measures" is arbitrary dosing with hormones of various types. What service does such therapy perform if it permits conception in a poorly fed mother by a poorly fed father? The forces that affect the fetus do not operate in women alone and do not operate only *after* conception has taken place.

One can't make promises that improved nutrition will create fertility in a barren marriage, but neglecting it certainly is prejudicial, not only to reproducing, but to the welfare of the baby.

Reproduction rests ultimately on all the essential nutrients in a good diet. There is one nutritional factor that years ago was reported to help previously infertile women to conceive after five years or more of failure. This is para-aminobenzoic acid, or PABA, which is sold in most health food stores. The endocrinologist who employed PABA gave 200 mg. daily to twenty-two women with long-standing infertility, twelve of whom had successful pregnancies within two years. PABA is no panacea and certainly should not be employed until both partners have been thoroughly checked medically. The reason for that admonition will not be apparent unless you realize that nature sometimes blocks impregnation for the reason that the ovum or the sperm is in some way abnormal, threatening miscarriage or, worse, the birth of a defective baby.

The following is a diet that was thoroughly tested in 1,000 pregnancies. Given its ability to help to bring a healthy baby into the world, the same diet can and should be used by both partners, beginning—I should hope—six months before conception is attempted. Following birth, with the mother nursing the baby, I suggest the diet be continued, with its supplements, to support lactation and to help the mother recover from pregnancy and nurse the child.

Daily Diet for Would-be Mothers and Fathers (Also to Be Used Later in Pregnancy and Lactation)

Eight ounces of unstrained, fresh-squeezed fruit juice, preferably citrus.

One serving of fresh fruit, *peeled*. Pesticide residues must be minimized.

Two cups of cooked vegetables, undercooked rather than overcooked. Cooking water should be saved and used to make gravies, or mixed with carrot juice as a beverage. To minimize amount of water saved, it can be boiled down rapidly in a shallow skillet.

One cup of salad made with dark green leafy vegetables, thoroughly washed. Dressing of vegetable oil. Do not use oils containing partially hydrogenated fat, BHA or BHT, or other artificial preservatives. Season as desired. Note: Intake of vegetable oil should not exceed five teaspoons daily. One teaspoon of wheat germ oil, which helps reproduction, may be mixed with other salad oil. Be sure to keep all oils refrigerated and thoroughly sealed.

Three squares of butter. Note: Do not use margarine, since it contains partially hydrogenated fat.

One serving of oatmeal, or whole wheat or other whole grain cereal, plus one teaspoon wheat germ and one tablespoon coarse bran.

Two eggs. If bacon or beef fry are added, be sure to buy health food store brands that do not contain nitrites or nitrates.

Six ounces of lean meat, fish, or fowl, with emphasis on liver, kidney, sweetbreads, and other organ meats. More fish should be served than is customary in American diets. This is particularly important if the woman has, prior to her pregnancy, been taking the birth control pill.

Four slices of whole wheat, whole rye, or whole corn bread. This does not mean commercial rye bread, which is white bread, nor pumpernickel, which is commercial rye bread with an artificial "suntan" (caramel color).

Conventional spaghetti, macaroni, and noodles should not be

used. Use high-protein pasta products, made with added soy flour and wheat germ. Brewer's yeast, wheat germ, and nonfat dried skim milk can be added to appropriate recipes.

For dessert, whole gelatin desserts (made at home from whole, unflavored gelatin with added fruit); stewed fruit, fruit whip, yogurt; * home-baked cakes, cookies, muffins, etc., made from whole grain or from unbleached white flour, with a teaspoonful of wheat germ (not defatted) per cup of flour.

Supplements for both partners in the preconception period differ from those in pregnancy only by the extra PABA taken before conception. The supplementary amount for the woman is 200 mg. daily; for the man, 100 mg. The supplements include a low-potency multiple vitamin-mineral, B complex, and vitamin E concentrate. Vitamin E is always used in the form of mixed tocopherols, rather than alpha tocopherol alone. The potency is 100 I.U. daily. A handful (literally) of coarse miller's bran is used by each partner daily. This can be added to cereal, yogurt, or baked products, waffles, and pancakes. Remember in the flour foods to use a teaspoonful of wheat germ to each cup of flour, particularly important if the flour is white (and unbleached).

When pregnancy is confirmed, a half-dozen tablets of brewer's yeast or desiccated liver are added to the supplements, and the PABA discontinued, though there may be a small amount in the multiple or B-complex concentrates, which is not objectionable. If the unstrained fruit juice and fresh fruits are not being consumed, or not consumed in recommended amounts, 1,000 mg. bioflavonoids, preferably of citrus origin, should be added during pregnancy.

This regimen, meaning both the menu and the supplements, should be continued during lactation.

Should morning sickness be more severe or protracted than

---

* Yogurt can be inexpensively made at home, since the commercial product represents buying milk at more than $5 per gallon. A yogurt hotplate is inexpensive since it is nothing but a low-temperature warmer. Whole or nonfat milk can be inoculated with any good commercial yogurt and allowed to ferment into yogurt. Do not buy flavored yogurts, which often have many additives and are high in sugar calories. If you must sweeten yogurt, use a little honey, which has the virtue of being sweeter than sugar, allowing you to use less. Fruit flavor can be added with a teaspoonful of preserves per cup of yogurt. This food is an excellent snack for the mother-to-be.

usual, consult the physician about increasing the intake of vitamin B_6 (pyridoxine). This sometimes relieves the nausea. Another helpful device is to eat small, frequent meals, and in that framework, to separate liquids from solids, i.e., not to combine them in a single meal.

One important note remains. Most women anticipate "stretch marks" as an inevitable price for pregnancy. Obviously, this is more average than normal, since some women escape. Stretch marks are sometimes more of a price for inadequate nutrition than actual stretching of the skin. They are sometimes attributable to a zinc deficiency, created by the unborn's great need for the nutrient, thereby depriving the mother. In the multiple mineral supplement, zinc is usually, and should usually, be included. A dose of 15 mg. daily would be a protective supply.

INSOMNIA

Insomnia can be a deceptive term, especially when used by the aged. They will vow that they had little or no sleep, a complaint to which the physician responds with sleeping pills, sometimes in doses that are excessive for the elderly, for an old body metabolizes drugs much more slowly than a young one. It is said that breaking down a drug takes an hour longer for each year of adult life, meaning that a thirty-year-old disposes of the medication in thirty hours, while the seventy-year-old may need nearly three days. Often, the aged sleep more than they realize, not only at night, but in unrealized catnapping by day. There is also the fact that less sleep is normally required as one grows older; in fact, in individuals whose sleep requirement does not diminish, or actually increases, there is statistically a greater risk of a stroke.

The amino acid tryptophane has been found to reduce sleep latency—that time between settling down to sleep and actually doing so. Taking 500 mg. of tryptophane at an early evening hour has been found helpful. Higher doses are used but should be medically supervised. It is believed that the effect comes from conversion of tryptophane into a neurotransmitter, serotonin, which we know to be a "calming" brain chemical. If it does, vitamin B_6 (pyridoxine) and niacinamide should help. Serotonin, incidentally, is also supplied by walnuts, tomato, and banana. It was thought that the proverbial glass of hot milk before retiring was helpful because of the high tryptophane content. This is not so, for to yield maximum effect, amino acids must be taken singly; otherwise, they compete with each other for entrance to the brain. It is more likely that the calcium in milk, which reduces neuromuscular irritability, is responsible for the effect.

There are other nutrients with a quieting and sometimes almost a tranquilizer effect. Inositol has such an action, as does vitamin E, which long ago was identified as dampening the transmission of anxiety.

Ordinarily, inositol is associated with vitamin B complex and it would be recommended that the group be taken together. However, the vitamin B complex contains factors that stimulate some individuals, an effect that may be an advantage early in the day, but certainly not at night. Label doses of inositol and of vitamin E may be too low.

I previously noted that vitamin B_6 tends to increase the vividness and your memory of your dreams. This action, if the dose is too high, can interfere with sleep, which is another reason for insomniacs to avoid the use of the vitamin B complex at night.

LACTOSE INTOLERANCE

There are many individuals—most of them adolescents or adults, some of them younger—who do not tolerate milk. The intolerance was misinterpreted as allergy for many years, until it was realized that lack of an enzyme, lactase, needed to break down milk sugar (lactose), was responsible for the difficulty. If lactose reaches the bowel without prior normal digestion (enzymatic breakdown), the bowel bacteria attack this simple sugar, and the result is cramps, diarrhea, and flatulence. Jews, blacks, and Orientals are particularly subject to lactase deficiency in adulthood.

There are three resources available to the lactase-deficient. One, of course, is avoidance of milk and milk products containing lactose. In some individuals, the problem is related to amount, meaning that they will tolerate small quantities of these foods without disturbance. In others, it is so severe that they must totally avoid lactose. In still others, for reasons not completely understood, milk products containing lactose are tolerated *if they are taken in forms other than ordinary cow's milk*—as yogurt, for example. This is also true of some people with actual milk allergy. Occasionally available in the health food stores is the enzyme lactase, which theoretically should solve the problem, but the reports I have had are mixed. The enzyme supplement is at least worthy of the trial.

Many cheeses contain too much lactose for those with little tolerance. For their benefit, I am supplying a list of cheeses that contain less than 0.5 percent lactose. These in reasonable quantities should be tolerable.

American Kraft cheese
American Red cheese
Bel Paese
Bondon
brick American
Brie, French
Caciocavallo, Italian
Camembert, French
Cheddar, Canadian
American Edam
Holland Gouda
German Limburg
American Mysost
Italian Parmesan
provolone
ricotta, Italian
Stilton, English

MÉNIÈRE'S SYNDROME AND TINNITUS

Ménière's syndrome includes ringing or other noises in the ear, loss of hearing in some degree, and dizziness that is often incapacitating. The symptoms have not been successfully treated medically, which is understandable, for the problem has been approached as if it involved only the ear and the semicircular canals that control the sense of balance. Actually, Ménière's is usually a result of metabolic disturbance, involving the whole organism and very frequently centered in carbohydrate metabolism. Abnormal "management" of starches and sugars is frequently the key. The most common form of this disturbance is hypoglycemia, and I have seen Ménière's disappear when carbohydrate metabolism was controlled with a low blood sugar diet. Frequently, hypoglycemia isn't present, but elevated levels of blood insulin *are*. These can also cause the symptoms. The therapy is the same as for hypoglycemia (See page 93). I have also seen it controlled with a few grams of bioflavonoids daily. The important point is the realization that the trouble isn't in your ear.

THE MENTALLY RETARDED

As it has been said that in every fat person there is a thin person screaming to be released, so is there in the mentally retarded a potential that often is never achieved, and I prefer, as do some fine medical nutritionists, to look upon the mentally retarded as being mentally dormant, awaiting awakening. The philosophy is not based on wishful thinking. Dr. Henry Turkel, unrecognized, unsung, has been upgrading Down's syndrome children successfully for many decades, not only lifting them to a higher level of functioning, but even inducing physical improvement that frees them of many of the physical characteristics by which most of us recognize them as Down's children. He accomplishes this with a combination of nutrients, such as vitamins and minerals, hormone therapy, and medication. Ironically, the Japanese government recognized the value of his contributions and sent a team of physicians here to observe his work, whereas the American government—via the FDA—persecuted him on the grounds that nothing can be done for a genetic disorder—this, while he has serial X-rays that show normalization, and case histories (by the hundreds) of children, once pronounced ineducable, who are now able to care for themselves and to function in society, the family, and the work world. The treatment Dr. Turkel uses is complex and, of course, therapeutic, and requires medical supervision. I am therefore not describing it in detail, but in the Appendix you will find this physician's address. Perhaps you can persuade your physician to communicate with him in behalf of your Down's syndrome child.

It is anomalous, considering Dr. Turkel's lifetime accomplishments having been met with derision, cynicism, and denunciation, that headlines recently announced that vitamin-mineral supplements had markedly raised the IQs of retarded children, including a group with Down's syndrome. For some of the latter children, the rise was as much as twenty-five points—enough to take a child out of the imbecile and idiot class and into the retarded, or from the retarded to the slow learner class.

Down's syndrome actually represents a glycogen-storage disease. This is totally different from other types of retardation. Multifaceted, the disorder creates a slow-motion picture of a normal child, never catching up. Yet these children are markedly responsive to many types of stimulation. As an example, a famous dental nutritionist, Dr. Weston Price, stimulated pituitary function in a Down's child by widening the dental arch. The child gained a number of years in mental function.

Mental retardation of other types do not involve glycogen-storage disease and may not necessarily reflect pituitary inadequacy. Yet these children, too, may respond to nutritional stimulation of mental function. In this, there is no magic nutrient, no wonder diet. The basic nutrition must be excellent, which means not only a diet meeting the child's needs, but one free of gratuitous insults like preservatives, dyes, excessive sugar, and overprocessed starches. One would not want in such a child's foods the trans fats (see page 164), which may disturb the permeability of the brain cell membranes. The child has enough problems without adding nutritional insult to brain injury.

Under your doctor's eye, there is a wide range of supplements that, added to the good diet, may stimulate cerebral function. L-glutamine is an example. This is converted in the brain to glutamic acid, which is a stimulant to brain and nervous system function. (Glutamic acid itself was formerly used, but it is difficult for this to gain access to the brain. The blood-brain barrier (a filter which allows the brain to choose what it will from the blood) stops most of it, while L-glutamine, which is a related compound, readily passes the barrier.) Nerve transmission may be helped with the vitamin B complex, plus added inositol. Choline or high phosphatidyl-choline-lecithin may be used to raise the level of acetylcholine, a neurotransmitter that is stimulating and that may help memory. Appropriate supplements of calcium and trace minerals, the need determined by hair, blood, and urine analysis, may provide some of the missing links. I am not being specific for several good reasons: Doses must be equated to the needs and, obviously, to the age of the child. However, a start may be made with a multiple vitamin-mineral supplement formulated for children. These are available in liquid form for children who can't swallow capsules or tablets. They also are provided in chewable tablets with acceptable, natural flavors. Note: Such supplements should not be given by laymen to Down's syndrome children, for there is a type of vitamin D they tolerate and a type that is toxic for them. Added vitamin B_6 may be needed.

When brain injury is an entity in the problem, octocosanol can be tried. It has occasionally markedly benefited cerebral palsy children, improving both motor and brain function. This is available in a wheat germ oil concentrate, it being a natural component of that oil.

Information concerning dosage will be sent to physicians on request. Such information will result in treatment falling on infertile soil if you do not remember that supplements are not a license for poor diet. Improvement of the diet comes first. I suggest that you read Dr. Lendon Smith's *Foods for Healthy Kids,* a paperback published by McGraw-Hill, since detailed, long-term menus do not fit into the format of this text.

MULTIPLE SCLEROSIS

*P*hysicians caring for multiple sclerosis victims are well aware that the establishment in that field is more efficient in soliciting funds than in finding cures for the disease. I receive many inquiries from doctors who, frustrated in trying to help their multiple sclerosis patients, are earnestly open to suggestions. What follows is the text of a letter I send in response to such queries, with the technical language simplified.

Allergic (or maladaptive) reactions contribute much more to the symptoms of multiple sclerosis (MS) than has generally been recognized. So many of these patients are sensitive to wheat gluten, and a smaller group sensitive to milk, that I strongly urge sublingual or Rinbel testing for these reactions. Conventional skin tests will not necessarily reveal such an intolerance, and more sophisticated or different tests are likely to be needed. The *kinesiological* method, in which muscle strength is used as an indicator of illness or health, is often the easiest, but this isn't accepted as yet by the profession at large. All foods, chemicals, and drugs to which the patient is exposed should be tested. The Swank diet, emphasizing fish, is sometimes helpful. I don't believe this is predicated upon escape from saturated fats so much as it may be based on an intake of certain substances present in the fish. Both are fatty acids, one of which must be present in the myelin sheaths, and another is helpful in reducing blood viscosity and discouraging cholesterol deposits.

The diet itself should be served in frequent small meals, rather than the conventional three larger meals daily, with the fish replacing most animal protein. Sardines and mackerel are best.* The purpose is to exercise better control of the changes in blood glucose levels, since this relieves these patients of the stresses of sudden changes. Multiple sclerosis patients are notoriously sensitive to stress. The low-carbohydrate hypoglycemia diet is suitable, but the patient should be encouraged to experiment to find the optimal level of carbohydrate intake, which should be in the form of complex starches rather than simple sugars.

Complex carbohydrates are available in foods like starch vegeta-

---

* In lieu of high fish intake, capsules of marine oil can be used.

bles, whole grain bread, unrefined cereals, brown rice, bulgar wheat, beans, and whole wheat pasta; simple sugars or carbohydrates are foods like sugars of any sort and fruits. These cause a rapid release of glucose into the bloodstream, followed by a rapid drop. While fruit is a simple carbohydrate, the natural sweetness does not have the same effect on glucose levels as does refined sugar, but some prefer to restrict the amount of fruit anyway. The prohibition on milk and wheat should, of course, be observed if an allergic reaction has been identified. Rice cakes made from brown rice and rice bread may be substituted for wheat. A calcium supplement, preferably orotate, may be used to compensate for the withdrawal of milk calcium.

For many years, I have suggested to physicians the administration of a twenty-eight-carbon, long-chain, waxy alcohol, octocosanol, which I know to be markedly helpful in MS. I originally used it because it is capable of increasing muscle tone in these disorders of nerve and muscle; but it obviously has had other effects. This is known as the "neuromuscular factor" in wheat germ oil; it is known to help babies with insufficient muscle tone to move their heads, for example.

Octocosanol is available in two forms. It is concentrated in wheat germ oil to about five times the naturally occurring amount, and it is available in the health food stores as Prometol. The supplementary dose is one capsule three times daily. Experience has taught, however, that the oil content of this concentrate may not be tolerated well by some MS patients, causing diarrhea, which makes use of this form difficult, if not impossible. For such individuals, I suggest that the physician administer crystalline octocosanol, which is available in higher potency from the same manufacturer. However, since it is best in its natural medium, meaning in unsaturated fat, I try to accompany the crystalline substance with evening primrose oil. It encourages synthesis of a prostaglandin that, in turn, encourages circulation.

Evaluation of the therapy requires ninety days. If there is no response by then, further trial isn't likely to be productive. In that period of time, I have observed improvement in many symptoms, including vision, bladder and bowel control, ataxia, involuntary movement of the eyes, and, obviously, in handwriting. If the handwriting has been affected, this becomes a delicate method of evaluating progress, and often is a good technique for distinguishing between a spontaneous remission and a therapeutic response.

It is essential to accompany evening primrose oil with antioxidants, including vitamin E (in the form of mixed tocopherols), vitamin C, selenium, and lechithin. Therapeutic doses will be set by the physician. Supplementary intake of vitamin E, mixed tocopherols, measured in terms of alphatocopherol content, from 200 to 400 units; vitamin C, timed-release form, 500 mg. twice daily; selenium, 50 mcg. to 100 mcg. as supplied by yeast concentrate; and lecithin, two teaspoonfuls of granules daily. (Lecithin capsules should not be used. Granules may be incorporated in tomato juice or mixed with cereal if milk allergy does not interfere.) Supplementary intake of octocosanol is 2 mgs. daily. The physician may use larger amounts profitably, but more than 10 mg. is not likely to yield added benefit.

MYASTHENIA GRAVIS

Myasthenia gravis—grave weakening of the muscles—has long been considered a disease of unknown origin, involving a failure of the chemistry at the junction between the nervous system and the muscles. The treatment has been based on elevating the body level of a neurotransmitter, acetylcholine, though the evidence indicates that the problem is not so much in the amount of neurotransmitter as in insufficient or ineffective receptors for the chemical. Nonetheless, accepted treatment for myasthenia gravis rests on drugs that raise acetylcholine levels in the body. It is a procedure not without risks, because the drugs can, like all medications, prove too effective, raising acetylcholine levels too high. This creates what is called the "cholinergic crisis," a fancy name for a side reaction that can be deadly.

If raising acetylcholine levels to normalize transmission of nerve impulses to muscles is potentially helpful to myasthenia gravis patients, medical men should reflect on the way in which acetylcholine is derived in the normal body. It is synthesized from three nutrients: choline (a B complex factor); pantothenic acid, and, in the facilitating enzyme, manganese. When I first proposed this natural approach, which offers no danger of excessive yield of acetylcholine, medicine had not recognized that dietary choline is in fact utilized by the body. Now that it is recognized, it is time for medicine to take the second step and combine the nutrients to provide what the body needs to synthesize the neurotransmitter. Since this is purely therapeutic, I am not providing the dosage, but will supply information to your physician on request directly from him.

There is another dietary factor that may be involved in the origin of myasthenia gravis. The nightshade foods, described previously for their part in initiating or worsening arthritis (pages 10–13), work some of their mischief by interfering with acetylcholine metabolism. So far as I know, only one case of myasthenia gravis has been treated by withdrawing the nightshade foods from the diet. That was a severe case, crippled by the disease. According to the physicians at the Johns Hopkins Myasthenia Gravis Clinic, a muscle biopsy now indicates that the patient is completely free of the disease. Under your physician's management, it would certainly seem worth the trial. For, as I pointed out when discussing the nightshades' role in arthritis, no one loses by omitting tomato, white potato, all peppers (save black and white pepper), and eggplant from the diet.

Octocosanol has been discussed (page 24). This nutrient is classified as ergonomic, a term that translates as "aiding muscle energy." It would also seem worth the trial. Octocosanol is best used in its natural medium, which is wheat germ oil.

My experience as a consultant in myasthenia gravis is limited, but the benefits I have observed, considered in the light of the limited response to the drugs, and the dangers they present, urges a trial of the nutritional therapies.

MYOPIA

Rejecting innovative ideas in the ignoble tradition of medicine, ophthalmologists have long considered eye exercises to be much less rewarding than has been claimed by specialists in orthoptics. I have personal knowledge of the effectiveness of these exercises in myopia. Some twenty-five years ago, a foundation in the field of vision assembled a group of myopes from my radio audiences and carefully tested eye exercises, reporting a significant improvement in many of the near-sighted subjects.

In recent years, orthoptic specialists have expanded their armamentarium far beyond eye exercise. They now recognize that nutrition plays a role in improvement of the near-sighted. Specifically, they report that deficiencies in vitamin C and chromium are the critical variables in the development of myopia. Formerly, excessive use of the eyes for close work had been indicted. It appears from this late and largely unknown research that close work will not harm the vision *if* the individual is well supplied with vitamin C and chromium. Chromium is not utilized by the body unless it is organically complexed, as it is in yeast. For those under forty, 32 mcg. of chromium, in the form of the glucose tolerance factor from yeast, is the supplementary intake. This is doubled for those over forty. (If the individual is diabetic, the physician may wish to prescribe more. Caution must be observed when this is done with diabetics taking insulin, since the chromium glucose tolerance factor may lower the insulin requirement.) The range of vitamin C intake is 250 mg. to 2,500 mg. daily as a supplementary amount. Ideally eye exercises are coupled with the nutritional regimen. Sugar intake must be minimized.

NUTRITIONAL PREPARATION FOR HOSPITALIZATION

*F*asting is the hospital method of preparation for surgery, which will be accompanied or followed by intravenous "feeding" with glucose. Whatever the sound scientific reason for dosing a sick person with sugar by vein, the effect is that of physiological stress, for that is what excess sugar does to the organism.

Fasting is also practiced by the medical department of the hospital. A typical case is that of a seventy-five-year-old man, hospitalized in coma for bilateral lobar pneumonia. During nine days in coma, he was given glucose intravenously and injections of antibiotics. When asked why protein and vitamins and minerals were not administered, the resident physician remarked that the hospital administration didn't "believe in vitamins." The patient died on the tenth day. Question: If he had not been in coma, would they have starved him, save for sugar in his veins, for more than a week?

There is also the matter of hospital food. Though menus are compiled by registered dieticians, hospital meals, to put it mildly, do not encourage patients to eat. One reason can be found in the advertising in the food technology journals to which dietitians subscribe. A typical headline reads: "Dessert—1½¢ per Portion." It tastes like it, too.

These practices impose poor nutrition on sick people whose dietary history certainly didn't contribute to maximum well-being. Surveys of American dietary habits invariably turn up large groups whose menus are inadequate sources of factors important to the immune system, to the glands that must resist stress, and to healing. Yet the relationship between your nutritional habits and your chances of recovering from an illness severe enough to require hospitalization is direct. I am saying that your past menus very much determine whether you will have complications and whether, indeed, you will recover.

A recent survey tells the story. In it, two admittedly incomplete tests allowed physicians to predict recovery or disaster. The tests included serum albumin and absolute lymphocyte (white blood cell) counts. The results will give you a good reason *now* to eat as if you knew that in the near future, you might be hospitalized for a *severe* illness. These were the findings:

1. If the albumin level was not above 3.5 grams per deciliter, there was a fourfold increase in complications and a sixfold increase in deaths, compared with patients whose level was higher.

2. When the white cell count (total) was less than 1,500 per cubic millimeter, deaths were higher by a factor of *twenty*.

When patients relegated to the intensive care unit of the hospital were thus studied, it was clear that low albumin values appeared in this group three to six times more frequently. Low levels in both tests were six to eleven times more frequent in the intensive care group. They paid the price for these markers of poor dietary habits, for there was up to a twofold increase in complications and four times as many deaths in those who flunked these tests as compared with those who passed.

It is surely obvious that it would be a good investment to have your physician check these two parameters—the serum albumin and the absolute lymphocyte (white blood cell) count now, while you're well. The blood chemistries taken in the ordinary "complete" physical should cover them. Should you fail to pass, you ought to check your protein intake—from meat, fish, fowl, eggs, milk, cheese, and dried peas and beans, to be sure that you are obtaining at least half your body weight in grams of protein. Any book of food charts will give you the needed data for diet analysis, and there are computer facilities your physician can call upon, if you prefer. To this precaution, you add the use of a multiple vitamin-mineral supplement, a B-complex concentrate, and at least an additional 250 mg. of vitamin C daily. In this way, you ensure your intake of the factors that build the white blood cells and create the serum albumin, as well as those, like vitamin C and zinc, that are critical in healing.

NUTRITIONAL PROBLEMS OF THE ELDERLY

*T*he nutritional sins of youth and middle age are paid for in old age. Not only is it intrinsically difficult to repay the penalties for a lifetime of inadequate nutrition, but the problem is complicated by failing digestive efficiency in older people. Some of the aged have insufficient stomach (hydrochloric) acid. Some have inadequate production of the pancreatic enzymes that are responsible for a major part of the digestion. These problems tend to hide in the shadow of the degenerative diseases associated with (but not caused by!) aging. To the arthritic elderly, however malnourished, *the* problem is the arthritis; diabetes, or a disorder of circulation or the heart, or Parkinson's syndrome receives the attention. Seldom do the patients realize that improvement in nutrition is the real priority, not only for the repair it may offer in the disease process, but even in responding to (and certainly in tolerating) the potent medications they swallow.

Your physician can now measure hydrochloric acid production

without the torturous procedure of yesteryear. You swallow a capsule that contains a small radio transmitter, the wavelength of which changes in accordance with the amount of acid present in the stomach. If you need hydrochloric acid, the physician can prescribe it for you, glutamic acid hydrochloride being one form. It should not be taken except on prescription.

Appraisal of enzyme activity is difficult and costly. I choose to assume that the aged system needs support, which is available in enzymes that can be taken by mouth. There are the papaya and pineapple (bromelin) enzymes, which assist in the utilization of protein. There are supplements of pancreatic tissue, supplying enzymes helpful in utilizing fats, proteins, and carbohydrates. Vitamin B_{12} absorption can be helped by use of the sublingual lozenges, discussed on page 22. Vitamins can be given by injection, to detour the inefficient digestive tract and raise enzyme production. This allows better utilization of supplements taken by mouth. These should include the multiple vitamin-mineral and B-complex supplements, of the type frequently discussed in this text. It is mandatory that, within the limits set by lifetime habits, the diet be improved as much as possible. Simple sugar (sucrose, honey, molasses) should be restricted as much as possible, and complex carbohydrates (whole wheat bread, whole grain cereals) substituted. Protein should be adequate, but not elevated until the hydrochloric acid and enzyme problems have received attention. Difficulties created by missing teeth and ill-fitting dentures must be realistically recognized. Food can be soft without being junk food. A bland cereal can be fortified with wheat germ. A hamburger can be improved with a little liver ground into it. Brewer's yeast and wheat germ can be added to pancakes, waffles, cupcakes, and homebaked bread. A reasonable amount of vegetable juices can be used to supplement inadequate intake of salads and vegetables, and some bran could be judiciously introduced to compensate for missing fiber. Adele Davis's text *Let's Cook It Right* and my own cookbook *(Carlton Fredericks's Cookbook for Good Nutrition:* New York, Grossett & Dunlap) are examples of sources for guidance.

What I am about to write should not be addressed to the elderly, but to those who would like to defer the toll of aging. If you think it's coincidence that Bob Cummings and Gloria Swanson, in ripe old age, look and act as young as they do, don't bother reading this. If you're receptive, consult the list of antioxidants that I discuss in relation to breast cancer (see page 139), and realize that antioxidants are not only anti-irradiation and anticancer; they are also anti-aging, and I know whereof I speak, for I have used them personally for many years. To the list of vitamin E, vitamin C, selenium, lecithin, sulfur-containing proteins (eggs), vitamin B_{12}, and vitamin A, add para-aminobenzoic acid (PABA). Coupled with a good diet, these supplements, even in the modest label dosages, will offer the chance to retain the prime of life, extending it far beyond the fifties and sixties. And don't be startled if gray hair recolors. It does happen on occasion, and it symbolizes the whole process.

NUTRITIONAL SUPPORT FOR WOMEN

- *PREMENSTRUAL SYNDROME*
- *DIFFICULT MENSTRUATION*
- *CYSTIC BREAST DISEASE*
- *UTERINE FIBROID TUMORS*
- *ENDOMETRIOSIS*
- *BREAST CANCER*

Male chauvinism becomes an art when the dominantly masculine medical profession approaches the problems of women.

If menopausal symptoms weren't available to "explain" the troubles of the middle-aged woman, gynecologists would probably have made it illegal for any female over thirty-five to visit a physician without a note from her psychiatrist.

Some menstrual troubles are "solved" with the birth control pill, though the troubles from the pill itself are not so easily solved. In lieu of that, the profession can always suggest that premenstrual symptoms and menstrual cramps are really problems of virgins, to be solved by marriage; and if that doesn't prove therapeutic, the next prescription is having a baby. Which leaves a hysterectomy and oophorectomy (removal of uterus and ovaries) as the last resort. Or experimental treatment with prostaglandins.

Prevention of breast cancer is simple, for surgeons. You just perform a bilateral mastectomy on women, in the name of prevention, even if they don't have breast cancer. The philosophy is primitive, but one must admit that it's difficult to have breast cancer when you don't have breasts. I know of one surgeon who performed the operation—removal of both breasts—on over a hundred women in one year. I know of another whose youngest patient to have both breasts removed was a child fourteen years of age. Her family history, he said, was so threatening that he congratulated himself on saving her life. (One might note that the term "family history" has no meaning. The history is relevant only when one knows who previously had breast cancer, whether in one breast or two, whether confined to the breast or metastasizing beyond, and whether before or after menopause.) An alternate suggestion came from an obviously sympathetic male researcher at the University of Texas: remove the breast tissue from newborn females. As simple to do as circumcision. He apparently didn't have time to arrive at the answer to the resulting problems—how deprived, for instance, would these women feel in not being able to give their babies the immunities and the closeness of breast feeding? He did suggest, though, that until the world is used to breastlessness, the women could wear pneumatic prosthetic devices, in essence, balloons for breasts. I am waiting for him to tell the women what to do when a lover is so stubborn that he can't be persuaded that balloons are sexy. I don't anticipate, though, that he would vote in favor of prostatectomies on newborn males, though prostate cancer is to men what breast cancer is to women.

An alternate method of preventing breast cancer, suggested by, again, a male oncological surgeon, is hysterectomy and oophorectomy for *all* women at age thirty-eight. From him, I don't expect the parallel suggestion of an analogous operation for all men to prevent prostate cancer: castration at age thirty-eight.

Before we detail what good nutrition can do in prevention or treatment of these disorders, we must decide whether women's troubles are simply the price they must pay for being feminine and for the biological birthright of being the bearers of babies. To rid our thinking of that ancient belief, I ask you to consider studies cited by an anthropologist, Lionel Tiger, showing that women who took examinations in college during their premenstrual week scored about 15 percent below their usual standard. Other studies indicate that nearly half of female admissions to mental hospitals occur during the premenstrual week. So do over 50 percent of women's attempts at suicide and nearly 50 percent of the crimes committed by women. Is that the normal impact of a process normal to women?

These symptoms, as well as the prolonged menstruation with heavy hemorrhaging, I long ago demonstrated are often a product of a hormone imbalance caused by poor nutrition. Over two decades ago, I devoted research to demonstrating the validity of that statement, my subjects being some 200 female students at a large university where I taught nutrition. To avoid the accusation of benefit from the power of suggestion, the students were not informed about the real objective of the experiment. They answered a long, preliminary interrogatory, in which, accompanied by many irrelevant questions, were these:

1. How do you know your menstrual is coming?
2. How long does it last?
3. Is the bleeding intense?
4. Have you had or do you have cystic breast disease?
5. Are there other members of your family with cystic breast disease?
6. Has anyone in your family ever had breast cancer?
7. Has anyone in your family ever had uterine fibroid tumors or endometriosis?

The subjects for the experiment were, primarily, those who replied that they knew their menstruals were coming because they "climbed walls," or terms to that effect.

In the paper I delivered, reporting this research before one of the holistic medical societies, the language of science doesn't reflect fully the flavor of the comments by the women who responded to the improved diet, some 70 percent of the group. The students who said the menstrual announced its imminence by making them "climb walls" remarked, after six months of better diet and the use of appropriate vitamin supplements: "I know it's coming, now, when it arrives" and "It takes me by surprise."

Other students also noted a reduction of other premenstrual symptoms, water retention, irritability, craving for sweets, nervousness, "drawing" pains in the thighs, and sensitivity of the breasts. More than half of the responders reported a shortening of the menstrual period from five days to three, permanently persuading me that five days may be average, but not normal. A few women were pleasantly astonished when persistent cystic breast disease improved and, in several cases, disappeared. One girl remarked to me: "As a man, you can't appreciate what it means to me to be able to go to sleep without wearing a bra." (The pain as she turned over in sleep had previously been great enough to awaken her.) In the entire group, there was but one student with endometriosis, who made no comment on her response at the time, but wrote to me years later to say that the condition had disappeared. She had waited to determine if that was coincidental, and decided it wasn't.

Uterine fibroid tumors are the reason for several hundreds of thousands of hysterectomies yearly. The following case history, one of many from my diary, illustrates the responses of some women to improvement in nutrition. The patient, a friend of mine, had been told by her gynecologist that a hysterectomy was needed because her tumors were large and causing serious symptoms. Familiar with my research, she brought it to his attention, and he consented to a trial of the nutritional therapy, warning her that the experiment must not be allowed to delay surgery too long. But when she returned for reexamination, he found that "vestigial buds" were all that was left of the large tumors.

Before I outline nutritional standards for women, let me confess that I have a hidden motive. It is pleasant to be the vehicle for information that helps physicians via harmless nutrition to treat fibroid tumors, menstrual disorders, and cystic breast disease. But the chemistry involved is also the chemistry of prevention of a common type of breast cancer. Since one women in fourteen will get it and prevention is, as usual, less salable than cure, I use improvement in the menstrual cycle and other lesser disorders to persuade women to adopt the type of nutrition that may prevent breast cancer. For one-third of all breast cancers are stimulated by estrogen (a female hormone), and the nutritional approach we are discussing is one that encourages the body to exercise stricter control over this dangerous hormone. It has been said that any substance that causes cancer in more than one species of animal is suspect for human beings. Estrogen causes eleven varieties of cancer in five species of animals, and while we eye the dangers of the synthetic hormone, prescribed for the menopause and contained in the birth control pill, we tend to forget that every woman is an estrogen factory, and the dangers of excessive estrogen activity are not confined to doses of the hormone taken on prescription.

Although the chemistry we are after is normal to the well-fed body, the responses of my students indicate that the well-fed American woman is rare. In essence, we are proposing, with nutrition, to help the liver to break down estrogen into a form that, while retaining its activity as a female hormone, loses the ability to overstimulate responsive tissues like the breast and the uterus. Specifically, we encourage the liver to convert estrogen into *estriol,* which has the great virtue of not being cancer-producing. In so doing, we decrease significantly many of the adverse symptoms of high estrogen activity. These range from premenstrual tortures to prolonged hemorrhaging, from uterine fibroid tumors to endometriosis, from breast cysts to encouragement of cancerous changes in certain tissues, such as the breasts.

The dietary changes needed are simple:

1. Adequate protein intake. This means half your body weight in grams of proteins. A 110-pound woman would thereby eat about 55 gm. of protein daily. For a reference, consider a portion of meat or eggs as providing about 15 gm. Other protein sources are used, including the usual fish, fowl, milk, cheese, and secondary sources such as beans and peas. Generally, we should try to have at least a small amount of animal protein in each meal.

2. Increased intake of the vitamin B complex, from whole grains, liver, and other organ meats, wheat germ, and brewer's yeast, augmented by concentrates of the vitamin B complex. Since estrogen is a fat-soluble hormone and we are trying to normalize its metabolism in the liver, we use a "lipotropic" B-complex concentrate, which means one well supplied with choline and inositol. This point is emphasized because many of these supplements, while providing generous amounts of the well-known B vitamins, contain very little choline and 500 mg. of inositol, or none at all. The supplementary amounts needed are 1,000 mg. choline and 500 mg. inositol in the recommended daily dose. If you already have a supply of a supplement that does not yield these quantities, you can add the use of a separate concentrate of choline and inositol, which are available combined and, in some instances, accompanied by methionine, a protein (amino) acid that is also important to liver function.

3. Reduced intake of sugar. This is critical; in fact, some improve-

ment in premenstrual symptoms, duration and intensity of the period, and cystic mastitis has been achieved merely by this one step.

4. Adverse reactions to caffeine and allied chemicals have been reported in some women with cystic breast disease. It is best to discontinue the use of coffee, tea, cocoa, chocolate, cola drinks, and those headache and cold medicines which contain caffeine. Peppermint, spearmint, and camomile tea may be substituted as hot beverages.

5. There are two vitamins that adversely affect women with high levels of estrogen activity. These are PABA and folic acid, the latter containing PABA as part of its molecular composition. PABA, which incidentally is not recognized as a vitamin, has the property of increasing sensitivity to estrogen; so does folic acid. It is, of course, a useful reaction for women who are at the low end of the estrogen scale.

When water retention is a significant problem in the premenstrual week or, for that matter, when one is on a reducing diet, vitamin B_6 (pyridoxine) becomes useful. This vitamin is not only a natural diuretic, and, as such, safer than the drugs used for that purpose, but it also stimulates the production of progesterone. This is the natural antagonist to estrogen.

Premenstrual syndrome, which is the blanket name for all the symptoms of the premenstrual period, is not listed, as cystic breast disease is, as a risk factor for breast cancer. However, I've long been convinced that the premenstrual syndrome and its usual accompaniment, the long cycle, frequently reflect a failure to control internal estrogen activity, and as such, are part of the "risk" picture. Heavy hemorrhaging may be also. In this context, it is significant to me that early menstruation and late menopause are considered risk factors for breast cancer. Both obviously imply prolonged exposure to the mischief-making hormone.

Accepted risk factors, other than cystic breast disease, include affluence (the woman with high income is at more risk), underactivity of the thyroid gland, and late pregnancy. Pregnancy before twenty-five is best; pregnancy after thirty is linked with increased danger. There is conflicting evidence on the role of breast size, some studies linking large breasts with increased danger, some pointing to small breasts. High animal fat intake, particularly from animal protein, has recently come under suspicion as a risk factor. I seriously doubt this, for the diets rich in animal fat in the affluent societies are also rich in sugars, which I know to be a culprit. In addition, the animal-fat theory should mean that Eskimo and Masai women should be decimated with breast cancer. They're not; and for many years, American black women, eating a diet high in animal fat, had less breast cancer than American white women, who ate less fat.

In the past, white women suffered more breast cancer than blacks, but the gap appears to be closing. Jewish women have been more susceptible than non-Jews. Obese women are more at risk.

Most of these risks can be reduced if not totally eliminated. That will not be accomplished by orthodox medicine, for it confuses early detection with prevention. Is not mammography exactly that? The Pap? And what is considered "treatment" for a risk factor like breast cysts—surgery—is actually treatment of a symptom, removing the end product of a disease process without affecting the process itself.

Apropos of my central thesis, which is achieving adequate liver control of estrogen, I suggest that you give thought to the implications of the use of Tamoxifen in the *treatment* of breast and other types of cancer on the reproductive system in women. Tamoxifen is an *anti*-estrogen drug.

Allergy in Cystic Breast Disease

There is a group of women whose adverse reactions to foods, chemicals, and drugs includes increased pain from cystic breast disease, as well as increased discomfort in the menstrual cycle and, indeed in the menopause (see page 142).

For convenience, we classify such intolerances as allergy, although they don't coincide with the definition of allergy as the orthodox practitioner in that field would give it. Actually, the language of Dr. William Philpott is more accurate: He calls these "maladaptive reactions."

Testing for such reactions is explained in the allergy section. Among many physical and mental effects of such allergic reactions, there may be a prompt worsening of the tenderness of cystic breasts. Since the body becomes "addicted" to the foods causing the trouble, it is often found that the food a woman prefers is the mischief-maker.

Since orthodox allergists do not define these reactions as allergic, they do not give the types of tests needed to identify them. Under "bioecological medicine and allergy" in the Appendix, you will find a means of locating practitioners who are aware of and test for these reactions.

The Thyroid Gland: Woman's Friend or Foe

There is an antagonism between the thyroid hormone and estrogen. When a woman suffers from cystic breast disease, disturbed menstruals, or uterine fibroid tumors as a result of excessive estrogen activity, the physician will frequently find the thyroid gland to be underactive. The American method of testing that function, however, raises some knotty questions when the underactivity is borderline. This is the question raised by individual differences in our chemistries: Is low normal thyroid function normal for *you*?

Conventional thyroid testing measures the amount of precursor of the hormone in the blood and the amount of hormone actually produced. At least one thyroid authority and many European physicians dissent. Such tests, they insist, do not measure how well the hormone is used by the body. Their philosophy is that one doesn't judge how a motor performs by looking at the amount of gasoline in the tank. One turns the motor on. The analogy in appraising thyroid function comes from recognizing that this gland is the thermostat of the body, and the obvious way to appraise its performance is to look at body temperature.

There are two requirements that make a temperature-thyroid evaluation valid. Obviously, the temperature must be taken properly. Second, whatever the results, they have no meaning unless they are associated with symptoms of thyroid dysfunction. To prepare for the test, a fever thermometer is shaken down as far as possible the night before. Immediately on awakening, the woman places the thermometer in her armpit while lying still. This is repeated on three consecutive mornings, starting on the third day of the menstrual, if she is in fact menstruating. If the reading averages less than 97.8° F. and she shows symptoms of thyroid underactivity, the test is regarded as positive—even if the results quarrel with the laboratory tests customarily administered.

Symptoms of thyroid inadequacy include feeling cold when others don't, requiring more clothing (or bed covering) than others do, catching frequent colds, dry skin, dry hair, brittle nails, constipation, fatigability, and easy weight gain. All the symptoms need not be present simultaneously.

If the reading is over 98.2° F., the thyroid is overactive, but again, this is not meaningful unless accompanied by appropriate symptoms. We are concerned only with the underactive gland (hypothyroidism), because of its effects in unleashing the ill effects of high estrogen activity in female disorders.

Two nutritional deficiencies contribute directly to thyroid underactivity. Most people know about iodine as necessary for the thyroid, but few know the full story. And still fewer know that vitamin B_1 (thiamine) deficiency in a degree far below what would be called a "deficiency disease" can cause irreversible underactivity of the thyroid.

The amount of iodine needed to support thyroid gland function is, according to orthodox nutritionists, minute—about one-tenth of a milligram daily. Yet there are studies indicating that there is a great difference in the requirements for different people. Human beings don't have uniform genes and biochemistries. The range may go from the "official" figure of 100 mcg. daily to as high as 1,000 mcg. (1 mg.). This is far more than the textbooks sanction; yet a University of Alabama researcher found a significant correlation between higher iodine intake and a higher level of health, in a study involving some 900 professionals and their spouses. With the current goal of reducing salt consumption, we are eliminating a large part of the iodine intake we formerly obtained from that source, and we really must seek additional supplies, if not from seafoods, then from kelp tablets or multiple mineral supplements that contain iodine.

One should not raise iodine intake appreciably without expert medical supervision, for there is a type of thyroid disorder that can be worsened significantly by too much iodine, and there are occasions when both the thyroid hormone and iodine are given. While every physician is aware of the effects of iodine deficiency on the thyroid, few of them know that thiamine deficiency, mild and chronic, can debilitate the gland irreversibly. The amount of thiamine and iodine in an average multiple vitamin-mineral supplement should suffice for preventive purposes; however, when therapy is needed, the physician may prescribe supplemental thyroid hormones. Dr. Broda Barnes, an authority on this subject, tells me that the synthetic thyroids that are medically popular are not as satisfactory as natural thyroid, such as is marketed by Armour and Company, among other sources.

We are left with two problems: What do you do when the temperature test says the thyroid needs help and the lab tests tell your physician that it doesn't? And how do you determine if you need, say, 500 mcg. of iodine daily, rather than the 100 mcg. the authorities have elected as a national requirement? The answers to both questions would necessarily come from a medical nutritionist. If he is familiar with Dr. Barnes's papers, books, and monographs, he is likely to trust the termperature test, and if familiar with the research of Dr. Emanuel Cheraskin, he is likely cautiously to raise your iodine intake in an effort to find your optimal level.

Two Nutrients Specifically Important to Women

Selenium: Anticancer Nutrient ☐ Selenium's role in arthritis has already been described. Because of the protection this mineral offers against breast cancer, women should realize that adequate intake of this nutrient should not be left to chance, because no woman can afford to speculate on two possibilities: (1) that she will not be the woman who will have breast cancer in her lifetime; (2) that her diet is an adequate source of selenium (or, for that matter, any other essential nutrient).

There are numerous areas in the United States where the selenium content of the soil is low. Supplements of the mineral or feed grown in other areas, richer in the nutrient, are given to livestock to protect their health. There are no government bulletins to warn women in those areas that a soil deficiency may make them members of the group of some 250,000 women who, at any given moment, are walking around with breast cancer and don't know it.

Eggs are now a good source of selenium, for the excellent reason that chickens are given the mineral to keep them healthy. Organ meats tend to be richer in it than steaks and chops. Whole grains, grown on soils adequate in selenium, are better sources than processed carbohydrates such as white flour, white sugar, white rice, degerminated corn meal, processed rye, and overprocessed buckwheat. One does well to buy whole grains, which usually means shopping at the health food store, though some supermarkets now have health food departments.

If there are many questions about the adequacy of the diet in selenium, supplements, preferably of organically bound selenium, from yeast, rather than sodium selenite, may be used in potencies from 50 mcg. to 100 mcg. daily. Therapeutic doses are described on page 21.

The dosage of selenium needed to achieve a satisfactory blood level in human beings varies tremendously. The margin between the selenium level of the healthy and the cancer-prone, while significant, is small. In healthy individuals, there will be from 20 to 30 picograms of selenium per 100 cubic centimeters of blood; in the cancer-prone, less than 16.

Vitamin E for Cystic Breast Disease ☐ For years the American Medical Association assured the public that vitamin E is adequately supplied by the American diet. This ignored a Tulane University study showing that a random sampling of the adult population showed abnormal blood fats that were oxidized (equivalent to being rancid), indicating lack of the natural antioxidant vitamin E. It also ignored the fact that Vitamin E is removed from the cereals and grains that comprise some 50 percent of the food sources of E in the average diet. It was at least a statement of ignorance concerning the practices of vegetable oil processors, some of whom remove the vitamin E, and sell it to the vitamin industry, to be resold to the public who buys the oil.

But the medical society eventually had to admit that vitamin E is useful for treating neovascular disease in diabetic eyes, in cortical cataract, and in benign cystic breast disease. It is to the last that I direct your attention. Rather than drugs with toxicity, rather than surgery, vitamin E (mixed tocopherols) can be used to treat cystic breast disease. A paper in the *Journal of the American Medical Association* reported favorable results with 600 I.U. daily. It is a report to which your physician is likely to give credence. The treatment can be added to the regimen discussed on pages 134–35.

Nutritional Protection against the Birth Control Pill and Estrogen Medication

Estrogen causes eleven varieties of cancer in five species of animals. This applies to the hormone regardless of its source—whether taken in the birth control pill, prescribed for the menopause, or, a factor that tends to be forgotten, produced in high amounts by the ovaries. You might remember that the original birth control pill contained high amounts of estrogen, and you were told that it was safe—which was a lie—and now you are being told that it is much safer because the estrogen content has been reduced. As I write these lines, I am reminded of four young women who died in a Michigan hospital on the same day, victims of strokes caused by the birth control pill that was "safe." When I asked an FDA official why the department had licensed a medication that could cause strokes and cancer, he replied that a slight statistical risk didn't justify barring the pill; but he didn't reply when I asked if he would be so complacent if he knew that his wife or daughter would definitely be the victim of that "slight statistical risk."

At the time, in the 1960s, I urged physicians to prescribe the vitamin B complex every time they prescribed estrogen, whether in the birth control pill or for menopause. That still stands, for some of the side reactions to the hormone derive from its effectiveness in inducing deficiencies in that group of vitamins and, not incidentally, in vitamin C. Users of the pill should supplement their diets with vitamin C, the B complex, and vitamin A, which really adds up to the recommendation so often previously made: a multiple vitamin-mineral supplement accompanying the B-complex concentrate.

Before discussing nutritional protection against estrogen side reactions in the menopause, let me note emphatically that I do not permit women in my family to take estrogen for *any* reason—birth control, menopause, menstrual irregularities, or whatever. There are other methods of contraception, none entirely safe, but safer than the pill; there is nutritional aid for the menopausal and for the victim of menstrual disturbances. But if I *did* permit estrogen therapy for menopause, I should choose a physician who knows enough to give progesterone with it, which is protective against the overstimulation of estrogen-sensitive tissues, like the breast and genitals.

But estrogen certainly would not be the first resource, for nutrition holds a great deal of relief for the menopausal woman. Even in the medical journals hopelessly wedded to estrogen therapy for the menopausal, there is sometimes recognition of its dangers and of alternatives in nutrition. The *Journal of the American Medical Association* is a good example. Queried by a physician who did not wish to prescribe estrogen for a patient with a history of breast cancer (surely an explicit recognition of the carcinogenicity of the hormone), *J.A.M.A.* recommended vitamin E as a safe substitute, indicating that it quiets the "sweats and flushes" for a large percentage of menopausal women. Which brings up the obvious question: If estrogen is dangerous for a woman with a history of breast cancer, why use it for any woman, when the chances are that she may be the one in fourteen whom the disease will strike?

The bioflavonoids, harmless nutrients of citrus origin, have helped many menopausal women. Calcium has been helpful; likewise, magnesium. The vitamin B complex has benefited many women in the midyears. Coupled with a good diet and a supplement of vitamin E, these nutrients have allowed many "change of life" sufferers to escape dangerous medication. But the time to start the nutritional procedure is long before the menstruals begin to fade. A more complete discussion of the menopause and recommended supplements is found in the following section.

Menopause, Osteoporosis, Atrophic Vaginitis

Beginning treatment of the menopause when the first flush or the first menstrual irregularity appears is a classic example of crisis medicine.

Treating menopausal symptoms with estrogen is an example of the risk-benefit type of medical thinking, except that you are the target not only for the benefits but for the risks.

Treating postmenopausal osteoporosis with estrogen and fluoride is another exhibit of risk-benefit philosophy, plus its being an obvious example of crisis rather than preventive medicine.

The time to deal with the menopause starts before puberty. The little girl who matures on a dietary intake of 300 mg. of calcium daily is much more likely to develop menopausal osteoporosis. If her intake is between 1,000 mg. and 1,500 mg., that risk is significantly reduced. A quart of milk yields 1,000 mg. calcium; four ounces of cheese usually provide that much. When she reaches the stage of discovering boys and, simultaneously, the importance of a good figure, and rebels against too many calories, a shift in part to a calcium supplement is in order. Since we have generous amounts of phosphorus in our diet, it is usually best to use a calcium supplement that does not contain phosphorus. This rules out bone meal and dicalcium phosphate, and suggests calcium orotate, which is a preferable form, or dolomite, or calcium gluconate. If sunlight is scarce, a fish liver supplement supplying vitamins A and D will be needed, though ordinarily, this quota will be supplied in the multiple vitamin-mineral concentrate I prefer to use. If the concentrate supplies calcium, it will not usually yield enough to allow the intake desired, which can then be achieved via milk products or another supplement of calcium.

Adequate intake of the vitamin B complex, as described earlier in the discussion of menstruation, is doubly important in preparing for the menopause. The woman whose diet does not make for a quiet nervous system is due to suffer more in the menopause with emotional storms. Lecithin, calcium, and vitamin E are also critical nutrients for her.

If you have not prepared nutritionally for the menopause and do not wish to be a target for estrogenic hormone therapy, all is not lost. A daily cup of ginseng tea, daily intake of vitamin E, and a generous supplement of bioflavonoids will reduce the intensity of menopausal flushes and sweats, and in some cases will wipe out the symptom. Do not accept the dogma that estrogen deficiency is *the* cause of menopausal symptoms. If that were true, all prepuberty girls and all men would have flushes. The concept that the ovaries are atrophying, producing less and less estrogen, and thereby causing the flushes and sweats is a lovely theory that is contradicted by the observation that some women who have had hysterectomies and still have their ovaries nonetheless experience postoperative flushing. Flushes start in the thyroid gland, and vitamin E helps because it is antithyroid, though not in a degree to cause troubles.

A dose of 400 units of vitamin E daily, in the form of mixed tocopherols, would be a good supplementary intake. Two to three grams of bioflavonoids daily, likewise. I prefer the citrus bioflavonoids, since they are more soluble, but hesperidin or hesperidin chalcone are acceptable, though usually more expensive. A B-complex supplement, as described in the section on menstrual problems, is helpful. And if you didn't protect your skeleton with adequate calcium intake prior to the menopause, you may already be on the road to osteoporosis, but a supplement of calcium will still be helpful—on the order of a gram to a gram and a half (1,500 mg.) daily.

Don't expect overnight results. Vitamin E often takes months to work its effects, though dividends from the other supplements may appear earlier.

Vaginal tissues tend to become dry and to atrophy after menopause, causing pain, itching, and difficulties in sexual intercourse. Women unwilling to take estrogen by mouth have often been persuaded to apply estrogen creams to the affected tissues, as if that were not equivalent to dosage by mouth. Actually, the hormone is readily absorbed no matter how it is taken. There is an alternative of which women are largely deprived because of insensate government regulations. A vitamin E ointment, or one containing both vitamins A and E, is quite effective as a treatment for most cases of atrophic vaginitis. However, FDA regulations would consider such an innocuous cream as a "new drug," and the manufacturer would be compelled to spend a fortune on research to back a new drug license. Such research, without the monopoly made possible by a patent, will never be done. But vitamin E creams are widely available and, if unscented, should be useful. The vitamin E potency of these creams tends to be low, but can easily be fortified by adding the contents of a few high potency Vitamin E capsules to the cream. There are also medical reports that vitamin E by mouth has been helpful, which means a double dividend since this nutrient also reduces menopausal flushes.

Constitutional Inadequacy

The diagnosis of "constitutional inadequacy" has unnecessarily blighted the lives of many women. These are women who complain of a sense of total inadequacy in meeting their responsibilities, however light. They suffer from sensitivity of the skin to tight-fitting garments, rough fabrics, woolen hose, and the friction of bras, garter belts, and panty hose. Their feet are usually heavily callused, without the excuse of long hikes or barefoot walking. They are therapeutically dependent on cola drinks, coffee, and tea, because they are always tired. They sleep so lightly that the slightest sound awakens them, or so heavily that they seem drugged, but awaken more tired than they were on going to bed. They are susceptible to sore throats, with the pain frequently radiating up to the ears, to bandlike headaches, and to poor circulation, particularly complaining of cold hands and feet. Their lovers think them frigid, but they deny this, pleading guilty only to a difficulty in expressing the warmth they nonetheless feel.

These women deserve a more accurate diagnosis, for their difficulties started before birth in inadequate development and function of the anterior pituitary gland. The clue is found in their palates, which are high and arched, with the result that the horseshoe shape of the upper teeth is compressed and the palate correspondingly narrow. This is not merely cosmetic, nor is it normal because it is average. The pituitary and the palate are formed from the same tissue, at about the same time, and interference with the development of one bespeaks possible interference with the development of the other.

The forces which narrow the palate are known. The process starts in the mother's pregnancy with a diet in which all the protein is well cooked, characteristic of the way we eat meat, fish, and fowl. Even dairy products are overprocessed, for milk is pasteurized and cheese often cooked to a uniform flavor.

It is not coincidence that pregnant animals fed exclusively on cooked protein often bear young with narrow palates. Primitives normally broad of palate will bear babies with narrowed palates if dietary protein is all cooked.

A second force in narrowing the palate is the passage through the birth canal, the human head having reached about the maximum size that the birth canal can accommodate. The third agency that causes a narrow palate is the use of the bottle instead of the breast in feeding babies. Widening the aperture in the nipple is a frequent practice when babies are having difficulties in feeding, and the child will repeatedly use his tongue to diminish an excess flow of milk. This, too, influences the shape of the palate. The net result gives us high, Gothic arched palates, narrowing the middle third of the face. It is a bonanza for orthodontists.

When these women are fed pituitary-stimulating nutrients, including polyunsaturated fat, vitamin E, PABA, vitamin C, and such trace minerals as copper, cobalt, manganese, plus zinc, they often respond with a normal sense of adequacy in facing their obligations, and mitigation of their other symptoms. A low-potency multiple vitamin-mineral supplement, plus label doses of PABA and vitamin E (as mixed tocopherols) added to a diet including uncooked protein, such as cheese made from raw milk and raw eggnogs, is worth the trial. The pituitary has, in these women, limited capacity to respond, and doses of stimulating nutrients will, if the potency is too high, increase rather than decrease the symptoms. This, of course, would call for lower doses or intermittent dosage—every other day, for example.

Lest anyone reject the thesis on the grounds that it singles out women, let me note that the pituitary deficiency in men, associated with the narrow palate, has a very different impact. If you wish to observe that, clip the news media pictures of men accused of crimes of senseless violence, and you will have a collection of narrow palates. This is not to say that broad palates never commit crimes of senseless violence, or that narrow palates do not mark respectable citizens. Your news photographs, though, will give you the food for thought that has preoccupied me for some forty years, though I have never been able to convince criminologists that there is a relationship between body and mind. Recent studies, though, have linked asocial behavior with diet.

Redistribution of Body Fat

What you are about to read, addressed to those normal in weight but with fat in the wrong places, is a chance observation. An obstetrician to whom I had suggested vitamin E as a nutritional tranquilizer for women in their first pregnancies noted that some of his patients who continued the use of the vitamin after pregnancy were able to redistribute body fat. The effects were particularly marked with the midriff bulge that often defies weight loss and also in the heavy upper arm and thigh and, occasionally, in the oversized bosom. With Dr. Harry Swartz, we organized a study of some 200 women with these common complaints. The nutrients employed were vitamin E (as mixed tocopherols), lecithin, and a high-choline, high-inositol vitamin B complex concentrate. Nearly one-third of the subjects showed a response, which in some cases was dramatic, since it involved areas that had not responded to exercise, massage, or reducing diets; in fact, many of the subjects were normal in weight, but, as they put it, had weight in the wrong places. An unexpected result was reduction of bust size in those in the 44–48 range; another was an increase in a few of the unendowed. An interesting case was that of a young model whose perfect figure was marred by a fat accumulation, resembling a half-melon, from the umbilical to the pubic area. This vanished, with no change in weight and no alteration of other dimensions.

This does not work for every woman. The percentage of failure is high. But there were other dividends. Some of the subjects found that the lecithin supplement had a quieting effect on the nervous system. Some twenty years later came the reports of the effectiveness of lecithin in improving brain function in the aged.

The vitamin E potency was 200 I.U.; the lecithin, two tablespoonfuls of the granules daily; B complex was high-potency, with 500 mg. inositol and 1,000 mg. choline in the daily supplementary intake.

In discussing these findings with Dr. Emanuel Cheraskin, medical nutritionist at the University of Alabama Medical School, I learned that he had encountered the same phenomenon of fat redistribution with a low-carbohydrate reducing diet. If the person is overweight, combining that type of diet with the supplements would be an ideal approach. (*See also* Infertility.)

OBSESSIVE-COMPULSIVE BEHAVIOR

*T*hose who are controlled by their behavior contribute disproportionately to the practices of psychiatrists. Their symptoms make this understandable, for they can't evade repetitive thoughts that interfere with making decisions, and they are captives of rituals, such as repeated washing of hands, walking only along certain routes, double-checking those decisions they can make, and indulging in repetitive questioning. Around these central symptoms may be depression, anxiety, and hostility. Anorexia nervosa is a variation of this kind of compulsion, in which the individual, usually a child or an adolescent, is driven into food aversion, which can cause actual starvation.

A clue leading to nutritional therapy came when medication that increases the brain-level of serotonin, which is a neutrotransmitter, proved markedly helpful to patients with compulsive behavior. Serotonin is manufactured in the body from tryptophane, which is a protein (amino) acid and also comes into the body in foods, such as banana, tomato, and walnuts. A major part of the tryptophane is converted into the vitamin niacinamide in the body. To discourage that conversion, and thereby increase the yield of serotonin, niacinamide is given with the tryptophane base.* Otherwise, the yield of serotonin from tryptophane would only be 3 percent, too low to be effective. All but two of the patients showed considerable improvement after thirty days of high dosage, and within six months to a year, "their conditions," said the psychiatrist, "were stabilized."

The two patients who did not improve were those with a history of aggressive behavior, which the therapy increased, leading to the warning that the tryptophane treatment should not be used in such cases. This is one of the reasons self-treatment should not be attempted by the layman. Another is that high doses of tryptophane are, according to the FDA, capable of causing serious side reactions. I have had no such reports from the numerous practitioners who have prescribed the amino acid, not only for obsessive-compulsive behavior, but to shorten sleep latency—the length of time between the attempt to sleep and the time that sleep actually occurs—nor were side effects reported when huge doses of tryptophane were given to help control the tremor in Parkinson's disease (see page 150).

OPTIMAL CARBOHYDRATE INTAKE

Establishing exactly the right amount of starch for an individual may be the key to weight control, increase in energy, or control of hypoglycemia. (Intake of sugar is theoretically easy: use as little as possible. No sugar in more than condiment quantities is desirable.)

The right amount of starch—the optimal carbohydrate intake for a person—is particularly important to those who can quickly gain weight by indulging in quantities of sugar or starch. Weight gain is a product of individual differences in carbohydrate metabolism. For some people, eating carbohydrates doesn't yield quick energy; it

---

* Vitamin B_6 is also needed.

simply creates fat, invites storage of water in the tissues, and promotes retention of salt. This combination of metabolic disasters makes it possible for such an individual to gain weight which is completely out of proportion to the number of calories consumed. That phenenonon is studiously ignored by nutritionists captive to the cereal–cake-mix–bread establishment, but was thoroughly explored and verified in a *Journal of the American Medical Association* article, "A New Approach to Obesity," in 1963. Just the right amount of starch—varying from individual to individual, is the key to successful weight loss and maintenance of proper weight.

The discussion of hypoglycemia (page 93) obviously invokes the same principle. Every hypoglycemic is an individual, and no standardized amount of carbohydrate will be optimal for each sufferer.

Where constant fatigue is the problem, with no disorder and no stress factors to explain it, the optimal carbohydrate intake may again be the solution.

Arriving at that level of starch consumption will seem simple, but may require the supervision of a medical nutritionist. The carbohydrate is completely removed from the diet—no starch, no sugar—and enough protein and fat, with a small amount of polyunsaturated fat to support reasonable functioning of the body, are consumed. Within a few days, a phenomenon known as "ketosis" will begin. This is the adjustment of the body to an unaccustomed problem: burning fat for energy, in the absence of carbohydrate. The usual symptoms, as this adjustment takes place, will be an increase in fatigue; but dizziness in mild degree, or headache may also result. At this point, carbohydrate is restored to the diet, beginning with small amounts—10 or 15 grams daily, equivalent to the yield of one slice of bread. The carbohydrate intake is then slowly increased until the symptoms of ketosis are gone. This is then considered to be the optimal carbohydrate level, and often promotes a heightened state of well-being, with better control of carbohydrate metabolism, and increased energy. In the reduction process for those previously described as mishandling starches and sugars, this level of carbohydrate intake promotes weight loss, particularly if the reducer is careful to include polyunsaturated fat in the diet, about five teaspoonfuls daily. This may be used on salads. Care should be employed in buying these oils, which should not contain partially hydrogenated fats, BHA, or BHT.

For the chronically fatigued without underlying disease or stress, there is another device in diet which is helpful, though it sounds too simple to be true: taking dinner at breakfast, and vice-versa. Energy metabolism is also stimulated by Vitamin B_{12}, which can be taken by injection or in under-the-tongue lozenges; and dessicated liver. The vitamin is used in supplementary intake of 1,000 micrograms in the under-tongue form, though the physician may inject more. Liver is a food, and there is no dose—a handful of tablets or capsules might be a rough estimate. (Don't buy the powder; it tastes like an accident in search of a victim.)

PARKINSON'S SYNDROME

Though drugs have been developed that relieve the progressive symptoms of Parkinson's disease, neither physicians nor patients are satisfied with the results or the side reactions from the medications.

Experimental treatments with amino acids (the building blocks of protein) have been helpful and essentially free of side reactions. The amino acids used, both essential in human nutrition, are phenylalanine and tryptophane. In the first trial, phenylalanine was administered to fifteen patients who had the disease for periods ranging from six months to thirteen years. The researchers stopped all medication for ten days and then administered a daily supplement of 200 mg. to 500 mg. phenylalanine for four weeks. Rigidity of the muscles was significantly relieved in eleven patients; walking ability showed considerable improvement in ten. Ten out of twelve patients with speech difficulties experienced satisfactory improvement. The symptom that responded most dramatically was depression, within one or two weeks of treatment. Side effects included only a temporary headache in one patient, lasting twenty-four hours, and insomnia in another, which was controlled by lowering the phenylalanine dose.

Tryptophane was used by another research group for the symptom that did not respond to phenylalanine therapy: tremor. They reported that twenty patients were given daily either 10 gm. by mouth or 6 gm. intravenously. In eleven of these, the tremors were described as satisfactorily controlled.

Because I strongly advise against self-medication at all times, and because there is an urgent reason for not attempting it with large doses of tryptophane, I am presenting some information that ordinarily would be written only for the physician. In it, the warning becomes explicit. Though I assume that the physician will wish to adhere to the dosages used by the original researchers, it should be pointed out that the dose of tryptophane may be unnecessarily large, and theoretically, could be reduced without impairing the effectiveness of the treatment. I mention this because there are reports that, though not confirmed, raise the possibility of adverse effects from high tryptophane intake for extended periods. If the tryptophane therapy increases the level of brain serotonin, which is a quieting neurotransmitter, and this is the pathway of its effect in Parkinson's, smaller doses would accomplish this if the physician discourages conversion of tryptophane into niacinamide, thereby increasing the serotonin yield, which nominally is about 3 percent. This can be effected by prescribing niacinamide with the amino acid and adding vitamin B_6, which is necessary for serotonin synthesis. Label doses of the two vitamins would be considerably increased for this purpose.

PERIODONTAL DISEASE

Contrary to the impression created by the fluoridation debate, the greatest loss of teeth rests on not tooth decay, but on disease of the gums and the supporting structures. Gum infection, pockets, malocclusion created by unreplaced lost teeth, and decalcification of the jawbone are the forces that combine to create periodontal disease, and too frequently, the process ends with dentures.

Traditional treatment has ignored nutrition and concentrated on eliminating infection, cleaning out pockets, removing plaque, and removing irretrievably diseased gum tissue. Indeed, there are dentists who to this very day stoutly insist that nutrition has no influence on periodontal disorders, a statement that could be justified only if the mouth had a circulation different from that of the body.

I write with conviction because I have been able to provide data to dentists that reversed the process of periodontal disease, including the loss of calcium from the jawbone. Needless to say, this isn't a panacea, and there are failures, but considering the discomfort, expense, and limitations of orthodox treatments, the patient is certainly entitled to this adjunct help.

The neglected evidence of the role of poor nutrition in periodontal disease is mountain-high. The purchase of irrigation devices like the Water Pik® to give the teeth and gums the exercise denied by processed foods is an example. Almost unknown to the profession and the public is an experiment, years ago, at the University of Alabama Medical School, which demonstrated that loose teeth (considered *normally* loose) tighten measurably after only a week on a low-sugar diet. Other studies at Cornell University and in Sweden clearly show that low calcium intake is routine in periodontal patients and confirm its role by marked improvement following the use of a gram of supplemental calcium daily for six months. Moreover, X-ray observation showed that the pattern of bone loss was reversed in a number of the patients, in whom new bone appeared.

Even in those in whom the process of bone resorption has inexorably reached its end and dentures are worn, nutrition still offers dividends which aren't usually utilized.

Denture failure is a source of unhappiness both for patient and dentist. In any survey of denture wearers, nearly a third say they are convinced tthat their dentures need refitting or that new ones are required. The sale of denture adhesives is a testimonial to such dissatisfaction, which is ironic, for the adhesives are believed by some dentists to increase the loss of calcium from the jawbone, making proper denture fit impossible. Since that bony ridge is indispensable to holding the denture, shrinkage in it, considered normal by some dentists, must ultimately make dentures unwearable. Yet that loss of calcium from the jawbone is inversely proportional to the calcium intake of the patient. Thus, good underlying bone is associated with a dietary intake of 900 mg. of calcium daily. Those with 500 mg. or less are in trouble. Actual measurement has shown that a supplement of 750 mg. of calcium daily, with 375 units of vitamin D, will reduce resorption of calcium from both dental arches by about 36 percent.

However, it isn't only calcium deficiency that makes mischief, but oversupply of phosphorus. The meat-potato-bread lover is not only calcium-deficient but high in phosphorus, so that the imbalance aggravates the deficiency; this is the typical candidate for bone loss with periodontal disease. Americans, because so much of our protein comes from sources rich in phosphorus and poor in calcium, have about two and a half times as much phosphorus as calcium in their diets. This is aggravated by our intake of phosphorus-rich cola drinks. This unfavorable ratio of phosphorus to calcium dictates calcium supplements that do *not* supply phosphorus. Bone meal may be useful for those whose phosphorus intake isn't exaggerated, but adds unwanted phosphorus for others. This explains my preference for calcium orotate, a supplement in short supply or for dolomite, a useful source also of magnesium, intake of which tends to be low in those who lack sufficient calcium.

Don't misconstrue the emphasis on calcium and magnesium. There are other nutritional factors important for avoiding and treating periodontal disease and bone resorption. After years of insisting that deficiencies of vitamin C or any other vitamin do not exist unless scurvy is present, the medical establishment recently admitted that you can be free of scurvy and yet have a vitamin C deficiency. Your tendency to periodontal disease may also be an example of vitamin C deficiency. A dose of 10 mg. of vitamin C daily protects against scurvy; it takes 2,000 mg. daily to protect the jawbone.

Niacinamide is obviously important to the health of the gums, as evidenced by the prevalence of periodontal disease in pellagra, even though the patients are remarkably free of tooth decay. Gingivitis (inflammation of the gums) that has only partially responded to vitamin B complex treatment will sometimes disappear when desiccated liver is added to the therapy. Sugar intake contributes not only to tooth decay but also to periodontal disease, for it causes elevation of blood cortisol, a hormone that has the unfortunate effect of causing calcium loss. While it has been recognized that vitamin B complex deficiency negatively affects gums, tongue, and lips, it is less well known that riboflavin deficiency can cause loss of the crest in the jawbone, directly contributing to loosening of the teeth. Even the problem of tartar accumulation is nutrition-related, for niacinamide has been shown to reduce that tendency.

If the diet is high in nondairy proteins (meat, fish, fowl, eggs) and there is a dominance of phosphorus, the calcium-only supplement should be used: 750 mg. of calcium daily is suggested. This may be reduced to 500 mg. if a reasonable amount of milk, cheese, yogurt, and other dairy products, excluding cream and butter, are in the diet. The usual multiple vitamin-mineral supplement is needed, as is a vitamin B complex concentrate. Extra vitamin E (mixed tocopherols) will be needed, since the quantity in a multiple supplement will not suffice. The supplementary amount would be 200 I.U. Vitamin C is best used in a timed-release preparation, 500 mg. morning and night, which achieves a more even blood level than large doses or ordinary vitamin C tablets. Extra riboflavin, to bring the daily intake up to 25 mg., will be needed. Desiccated liver capsules or tablets—a literal handful—is the day's supplementary intake, Brewer's yeast may also be helpful, a dozen or more tablets daily. If this dietary regimen is coupled with the necessary periodontal treatments, the best of both possible worlds is combined.

A treatment for periodontal disease has been suggested by the pioneer in prostaglandin research, Dr. David Horrobin. The prostaglandins are transient hormones—short-lived but very essential to the body, and produced as the needs of the organism dictate. When there is a prostaglandin imbalance, trouble is always the product. A common imbalance is too little of prostaglandin E_1 (PGE_1) and an oversupply, relatively, of PGE_2. This is held responsible for some of the joint inflammation in arthritis, for example, and may explain the responses to vegetable oil therapy in that disease (see page 25). Prostaglandin E_1 is manufactured by a complicated chemical process in the body, beginning with a fatty substance normal to vegetable oil—linoleic acid—and going through a series of conversions via gamma linoleic acid, dihomogamma linoleic acid, and, finally, PGE_1. This process can be interfered with by deficiency in the basic material, linoleic acid, or by deficiencies in insulin, zinc, magnesium, B_6, and niacinamide, by alcohol and by failure of the chemistry in the aging process. The trans fats—page 164—also interfere. The point at which the synthesis of the prostaglandin breaks down appears to be in the synthesis of gamma linoleic acid. Food sources of this factor to restore the synthesis are extremely rare. It is found in breast milk (not cow's milk), small amounts are in spirulina, and the only rich source, relatively speaking, is evening primrose oil. This is a costly material, but in aggravated periodontal disease, its use may be recommended by the dental nutritionist. Since it is a highly unsaturated fat, evening primrose oil administration must be accompanied with the biological antioxidants vitamin E, selenium, vitamin C, sulfur-containing amino acids, and lecithin, as well as the nutrients previously mentioned.

Correction of malocclusion, a "bad bite," and local therapy for periodontal disease take time. So does nutritional therapy. Once again, you must remember that it took years of nutritional bankruptcy to start or aggravate this mischief in the mouth, and it will take time to reverse it.

PICA (EATING UNNATURAL "FOOD")

Contrary to public opinion, food cravings rarely are an answer to the needs of the body. More often, at least in older children and adults, such cravings reflect a maladaptive reaction to the foods, which are "addictively" craved. However, when such cravings do reflect a need of the body, it is often not satisfied by the strange nonfoods eaten by those who suffer from a disorder called pica. This is in contrast to the eating of clay by pregnant women, which may represent an attempt to overcome a zinc deficiency. Such hunger for needed minerals may also drive children into swallowing nonfoods that may be toxic. A case history illustrating the response of such a child to appropriate mineral therapy is told by Dr. Allen Cott, an orthomolecular psychiatrist in New York City. He treated a five-year-old with a history of eating the nonedibles from the time she was mature enough to put things in her mouth. The pediatrician brushed off the worried mother's queries, assuring her that all babies put things into their mouths and they all outgrow the behavior. The mother pointed out that the child was swallowing the nonedibles, but she was still ignored. The baby began by licking the top of the Comet cleanser can, acting as if it were succulent. (This was a clue—there is a zinc salt in the cleanser.) She devoured candles, even though they made her ill, ate crayons and lipsticks and the graphite in pencils, Silly Putty, matches, cigarettes, and papers of all kinds. Taken outdoors, she ate dirt and sand the way other children eat sweets.

A hair analysis showed low levels of potassium, cobalt, manganese, and zinc. Elevated values were found for magnesium, iron, lead, and copper, the lead level high enough to be threatening. The child was treated with niacinamide, pyridoxine, ascorbic acid, vitamin B_{12}, manganese, zinc, and folic acid. Sodium alginate, an extractive of seaweed, was used to help to remove the heavy metals, such as lead, from her body. Some six weeks after the treatment began, the child for the first time asked for food, saying she was hungry.

At the end of five months, the parents reported that the child was dramatically better—she was less shy and had glossier hair and rosy cheeks. Learning improved, although the psychiatrist notes that she went through a period of four months when she was having letter and word reversals. Eventually the behavior disappeared. A follow-up hair analysis showed reduced copper and iron, and lead brought down to normal range. Manganese had increased by a factor of five, and zinc level was up by 40 percent.

While pica in this degree is, fortunately, rare, the history warns us that such behavior often has significant biological disturbances behind it. But they are treatable.

PRICKLY HEAT AND POISON IVY

It seems that medicine has forgotten the lessons taught when prickly heat decimated our military forces in the South Pacific in World War II. The remedy, discovered at that time, was vitamin C. It was taken by mouth in doses of 2 gm. or more daily, and it was also used in a water-soluble ointment form, containing from 3 to 10 percent ascorbic acid.

Folk medicine has used vitamin C similarly for poison ivy, augmented with local application of bruised plantain or aloe vera leaves. The treatment has been remarkably successful on occasion.

PROSTATE ENLARGEMENT (BENIGN)

Since prostate cancer is to men what breast cancer is to women, it is vitally important that men with symptoms of prostate enlargement undergo a thorough examination to be sure that it is benign rather than malignant. If the symptoms—urgency of urination, burning, reduced volume and force of urination—derive from the benign enlargement of the prostate, which is apparently part of the aging process, surgery may be urged upon the patient. If that suggestion has been made to you, be sure that you are an informed patient, which means that you must understand that the operation may leave some men impotent and may leave some incontinent, forced to wear the equivalent of a diaper. Add to that knowledge, this observation, which, unfortunately, has not yet reached the orthodoxy in medicine: Prostate enlargement has sometimes successfully been treated with zinc, in which that organ is extraordinarily rich; vitamin B_6, needed to help the absorption of zinc; vitamin E, which helps circulation; and vitamin C, which, with its diuretic effect, increases the volume of urination. Vitamin C is used in timed-release formulations, twice daily. The doses are on the label, supplementary, not therapeutic; and, as usual, the medical nutritionist may choose much higher doses. Those who respond to this therapy have sometimes reported virtual return to normal bladder function.

There is also a treatment unknown to many physicians but widely used by veterinarians for prostate trouble in aged animals such as dogs. It is a copper-zinc superoxide dismutase, administered by injection, and is, I am told by these practitioners, remarkably helpful.

PSORIASIS

There are no cures for psoriasis, thus far, in nutrition. The disorder is complex, involving more than the skin, and in some individuals, there is a strong emotional component in the onset of the disease.

However, the fortunate with psoriasis sometimes gain some relief from vitamin A and lecithin, supplementary doses, which, as usual, the medical nutritionist or dermatologist may considerably augment. Timed-release supplements of pantothenic acid have also helped. These nutritional aids should be discussed with your physician. They do not interfere with any other treatment in medicine.

Though I have not had the chance to observe zinc therapy for psoriasis, I have had reports of excellent response in some individuals. Zinc, of course, is indispensable in healing, but I suspect that its cooperative role with vitamin A is the pathway, making simultaneous use of the vitamin desirable. Supplemental dosages of zinc may be adequate, but physicians experienced with zinc therapy tell me that they have sometimes found it necessary to give truly large doses, though these are rarely required.

SENILITY

Demented, dehydrated, deficient, drugged, or deserted? It is easy to label a confused, disoriented, babbling oldster as suffering from "second childhood" from which there is no retreat. The facile diagnosis deprives the patient of possible help if his mental disturbance actually stems from unnoticed small strokes, lack of sufficient water, poor diet, side effects of drugs, or the emotional shocks of the loss of a spouse in a long-term marriage. These can stimulate or aggravate senility. The mistaken diagnosis pins the sole responsibility on the aging process, just as the symptoms enumerated by a forty-five-year-old woman may carelessly be assigned to menopause.

One would not suspect that mere shortage of water can mimic the effects of senility. However, exactly as the senses of taste and smell decline, depriving the elderly of the zest for eating, so may the center for thirst lose efficiency, and the older person then becomes dehydrated. One effect of this is a "thickening" of the blood, further impairing circulation (including that to the brain) that is already compromised by age.

Nutritional deficiencies in the elderly may almost be taken for granted. If poverty doesn't dictate an inadequate diet, the poor nutritional habits of a lifetime may. This is compounded by a lack of hydrochloric acid and a reduced production of digestive enzymes, which limits the digestion and absorption of foods.

The mischief that may be created by the wrong drug, overdosage, or improper mixtures of drugs isn't appreciated by the average family sheltering the disoriented, confused elderly relative. Often a drug useful when originally prescribed is used long after it should have been discarded. Overdosage results from patient error most of the time, but it may also derive from the nature of the drug. Digitalis, for example, is without peer for certain cardiac symptoms, but maintaining exactly the right blood level is difficult in some patients, and too high a concentration can cause mental symptoms that may be blamed on senility. Long-continued use of drugs to lower blood pressure can yield a Pandora's box of symptoms that can be easily blamed on aging. These diuretic medications (water pills) lead to the excretion of vital nutrients, which causes physical and mental symptoms. Compensation for nutrient losses is vital, and supplements are useful if competently prescribed.

An underlying disorder is easily missed in older patients. "Senile behavior" can be the product of many things: brain clot, anemia, underactive or overactive thyroid function, fluid accumulation in the brain, marginal kidney or liver function, chronic lung disease with a consequent deficit in oxygen supply, decrease in hearing, sight, or other senses, tranquilizers and other drugs affecting the brain and nervous system, diuretics, digitalis, oral diabetic drugs, painkillers, anti-inflammation drugs, sedatives, or excessive use of alcohol. Before the physician brushes off the conditions as "old-timer's disease," he must carefully investigate these possibilities.

Wrong combinations of drugs may be the result of incompetent prescribing, but the patient may arrive at these by continuing to use outdated prescriptions while also taking currently prescribed medications. In some instances, the elderly may be simultaneously cared for by two or even three different doctors, each unaware of the others' prescriptions. If a single pharmacy is patronized by the patient and his family, some protection would be offered, for the pharmacists, well educated in pharmacology, would be likely to detect drugs in collision and notify the physicians involved. This is one of the reasons for a recent proposal to license pharmacists to prescribe drugs after diagnosis has been medically established.

The emotional trauma of separation from a loved one or a change of living quarters and life-style can initiate or accelerate symptoms of senility. Interaction among the patient and relatives may itself aggravate symptoms of second childhood, which is to say that the aged person treated like a child slips more easily into the role. Experiments in treating the senile as adults, in a warm and accepting way, have resulted in more rational behavior, fewer symptoms of dementia, and even restoration of bowel and bladder control.

The entrenched dietary habits of a lifetime may have contributed to senile dementia, but though they may cry for revision, a head-on assault will earn no dividends. The "tea and toast to keep up my strength" habit, superimposed on a lifetime of poor dietary habits, now compounded by failing digestive efficiency and, perhaps, malabsorption of food, obviously must be changed. But those who attempt it must know what they are doing. For example, the protein intake of the elderly is often inadequate; in addition, the elderly aren't efficient in utilizing these foods and may need help ranging from vitamin supplements to digestive aids, such as enzymes and hydrochloric acid. While vitamin, mineral, and protein supplements often yield gratifying improvement in the senile, they are *supplements,* not substitutes for balanced diet. Zinc is not only essential to life, it helps maintain the senses of taste and smell, which are in trouble in many of the elderly. This is so specific that one can trace a relationship between the long-term use of diuretic drugs and diminished intake of foods, easily leading to malnourishment, which then masquerades as or aggravates "old-timer's disease."

In any event, changing the diet of the elderly is easier if changes are made in recipes rather than in the selection of foods. Nonfat milk powder can be used as an ingredient in custard, for instance, to compensate for other protein foods that have been rejected. Wheat germ can be added to all recipes made with flour—a teaspoonful to a cup of flour. About 3 percent liver can be added to meat loaf and hamburger; more would be likely to be detected. A limited intake of fruit juice can be offset by adding vitamin C (ascorbic acid), which, in powder form or crystal form, is easily dissolved. Brewer's yeast is another valuable addition to recipes, though quantities must be small until tolerance is exhibited. This applies also to bran. (See page 65 for the proper use of bran.)

Another problem of the aged derives from the mistaken concept that brittle bones and old age are inseparable. Very often, one hears: "She fell and broke her hip." Net result is often a wheelchair, sometimes for life, and sometimes successful surgery and repair. Few laymen realize that the sequence was actually the reverse: The bone broke and caused the fall. And still fewer trace any connection between brittle bones and being housebound and *deprived* of vitamin D from sunlight. Yet repeatedly, surveys have shown that even brief exposures to sunlight raise the low blood levels of vitamin D in the aged. There is a simple but often effective preventive measure:

old-fashioned cod liver oil and calcium in the diet, whether from dairy products or a supplement. Label doses are adequate supplementary amounts. Calcium supplements are mandatory—preferably preventively, before the condition starts.

Let me give you a glimpse at what a single vitamin did for a woman in her middle sixties. She was brought to a sanitarium, diagnosed as a senile dement, paranoid (with delusions of persecution), confused, and hostile. ECT (shock therapy) had been recommended, but the pyschiatrist had an intuitive feeling that the patient had not been competently examined for the possible physical causes of her behavior. He requested an examination at a major hospital. There she was found to be suffering from a vitamin B_{12} deficiency, which, while it had not yet caused pernicious anemia, had caused degenerative changes in the nervous system and brain. Treated with the vitamin, she became normal, the psychiatrist reported, reminding his peers that it has been estimated that possibly 1 percent of institutionalized "senile dements" might be rescued with vitamin B_{12} therapy. Whether his estimate is accurate or not, it should be obvious that nutrition offers protection for the aged, and nutritional therapies offer the chance of improvement.

While some of the aged may have gastric function efficient enough to break down hard tablets, many do not, and I prefer supplements in soft gelatin capsules or liquid form.

A multiple vitamin-mineral supplement or the two combined in one would obviously be a good investment for the aged. A lecithin supplement may be helpful, for the aging body grows less efficient absorbing fats and cholesetrol, as well as producing less of the neurotransmitter involved in memory. This is *acetylcholine*. Lecithin supplies a substance that is a precursor for this neurotransmitter. There is a type of lecithin three times as rich in this precursor as the ordinary kind. Called "high phosphatidyl choline," it can perform yeoman service for some elderly people, and on occasion rescues them from a mistaken diagnosis of senility. Vitamin B_{12} linguets, dissolved under the tongue, are useful. Of critical importance to the aged is a supplement of the vitamin B complex, which, in addition to the concentrated vitamins of that group, supplies a source of the natural, unknown factors, found in brewer's yeast, liver, or rice polishings. These factors are not available in the crystalline or concentrated form. As a good example, consider the "antifatigue" factor in liver. It significantly increases stamina and demonstrably has effects that are not conferred by any of the known vitamins, minerals, or protein of liver.

The B vitamins in the multiple supplement and those of the vitamin B complex supplement will overlap. This is calculated, for a generous intake is needed to offset the impaired digestive efficiency and absorption of the aged. To augment lecithin, choose a B-complex concentrate that supplies at least 500 mg. choline and 250 mg. inositol in the recommended daily dose.

Deficiency in vitamin B_6, important in the utilization of protein, is commonplace in most Americans and probably virtually universal in the aged. Moreover, this vitamin not only helps in the absorption of zinc, but aids the production of a hormone that aids circulation and helps to keep the eyes and mouth normally moist. Twenty-five milligrams of vitamin B_6 daily, including that supplied by the multiple and B-complex supplements, would be helpful to the aged.

If the older person's diet does not provide meaningful amounts of dairy products, such as yogurt, milk, or cheese, an additional intake of calcium should be provided from a supplement that does *not* supply phosphorus, such as calcium orotate or calcium gluconate.

Distributing the day's food intake in five or six smaller, rather than three larger, meals is a useful pattern for the elderly. It helps in control of blood sugar levels, blood cholesterol, and weight.

If cognitive functions are seriously disturbed, the medical nutritionist will begin vitamin therapy with injections rather than oral doses. This is calculated to break the vicious cycle of malutilization and malabsorption causing deficiency, and deficiency increasing malutilization. When he shifts the patient to oral doses, he is likely to prescribe very much larger amounts than those proposed in these notes for preventive purposes. He may also draw upon other nutritional therapies aimed at specific targets. For example, niacinamide, useful in the treatment of osteoarthritis, may be prescribed for an elderly person who is not arthritic, but has disturbances of the sense of balance. Octocosanol, a natural factor concentrated from wheat germ oil, may be recommended to increase muscle tone, so often poor in older people.

If cerebral atherosclerosis (hardening of the arteries of the brain) is actually present, all is not necessarily lost. Chelation can be used to try to improve circulation to and in the brain, and is often surprisingly successful (see discussion of chelation, page 83). Experience has taught me, though, that this technique should not be the first approach to the problem of the genuinely senile aged. Very often, the person who is thus demented has been malnourished for a long period before the deterioration of the brain became noticeable. Intravenous feeding, if good nutrition by mouth is difficult to achieve (or too slow), should precede chelation. The combination will sometimes restore a seriously demented oldster to normal brain function.

A distinction should be made between senility deriving from impeded circulation to the brain and that suspected to be caused by aluminum toxicity to brain cells (Alzheimer's disease). The latter disorder isn't related to age; in fact, it is notorious for causing devasting senility in relatively young people, apparently out of the blue. Treatment of this type of senility is a journey into the unknown, for much will depend on the degree to which important nerve cells have been damaged. The medical nutritionist may, in the absence of a diagnosis, attempt to cover both eventualities—cerebral atherosclerosis and aluminum-induced brain degeneration by treating the patient with choline, lecithin, magnesium, zinc, vitamin B_6, manganese, and brewer's yeast, plus egg yolks to supply needed sulfur-containing amino acids. To this list, if Alzheimer's disease is a possibility, I should recommend that the nutritionist add octocosanol, for my experience, though in less severe types of brain damage, indicates that this nutrient does what the neurology textbooks state as impossible: It stimulates the repair of cerebral neurons (nerve cells).

TEMPEROMANDIBULAR JOINT DYSFUNCTION (TMJ SYNDROME)

When missing teeth are not replaced, other teeth move to fill the gap. In moving, they may tilt, and the result is malocclusion, which the layman calls "a bad bite," It seems little known to the public that this apparently simple problem is very complicated and that it can cause symptoms throughout the body, ranging from severe pain in the face to pain in the ears, from headaches to symptoms of a gastric ulcer (which isn't there.) Merely reshaping the teeth, now an outmoded practice, will not solve the problem if it is severe and of long standing, for the jawbones and muscles have had to adjust to the improper bite and may not willingly go back to normal when the bite is corrected. Mouth appliances are necessary to relieve the symptoms by readjusting the jawbones and the muscles.

All this comes up in a book dedicated to nutrition because many sufferers with TMJ syndrome also have hypoglycemia. The coincidence of low blood sugar with this condition is believed to be meaningful. The conclusion? If you have been told you have TMJ syndrome, see page 96 for the self-test for hypoglycemia. If you flunk the test, you may profit greatly with a glucose tolerance test, for treatment of hypoglycemia is mandatory if you wish to recover fully from TMJ syndrome.

TRANS FATS: MISCHIEF MAKERS IN A HUNDRED DISORDERS

When fats are partially hydrogenated, food products result that contain much larger percentages of these unnatural fats than do natural, unprocessed foods. These fats interfere with the normal permeability of the cell membranes, which can lead to biological chaos and initiate or aggravate dozens of disorders. The trans fats also interfere with the synthesis of a fleeting hormone, normal to the body and ordinarily produced as needed, called prostaglandin E_1. This hormone has an indispensable series of roles in the body, and deficiency in it can contribute to atopic eczema, arthritis, cystic mastitis, menstrual cramps, tendency to weight gain, and elevated blood cholesterol and blood pressure; and that is a partial list.

To avoid excessive intake of trans fats, one *must* read labels. The revealing term is "partially hydrogenated." This guarantees an excessive intake of this unnatural type of fat—unnatural in terms of quantity present, for the trans fats do appear in some natural fats, but in nowhere near the concentration presented to us in the processed foods. Vegetable oil, margarine, cookies, crackers, cereals, and a thousand other staple foods are, unfortunately, likely to contain trans fats by virtue of the manufacturer's use of partial hydrogenation. His purpose is shelf life. My concern is your life.

Following is a list of common foods and their transfat content. Generally, you can minimize your intake of such fat by the precaution of label reading I've already suggested, but the red flag should go up when the following foods are on your shopping list.

Percentages were found to be:

> animal fats, 0.3–6.6
> breads and rolls, 0.2–27.9
> breadings and fried cursts,
> 12.1–33.5
> butter, 3.1–3.8
> cake, 0.4–24.0
> candy, 3.2–38.6
> cookies, 2.4–37.4
> crackers, 2.8–31.6
> French fried potatoes, 4.6–37.4
> frosting, 11.6–32.7
> margarine (stick), 17.4–36.0
> margarine (soft/tub), 10.6–21.3
> margarine (diet), 13.7–17.9
> mayonnaise and salad dressing,
> 4.5–4.6
> nondairy creamers and
> toppings, 0.4–13.7
> oil, 0.4–13.4
> pastries, pies, and doughnuts,
> 0.6–34.6
> pudding, 30.5–36.1
> shortening, 13.0–37.3
> snack chips and pretzels, 0.8–
> 33.4

PEPTIC ULCER

*Myths about diet for stomach ulcer have dominated medical treat*ment of the disorder. The emphasis on milk and a bland diet is predicated upon its "soothing" effect or its famed ability to reduce excessive stomach acidity; but in fact, both the bland diet and milk may have the opposite effect. Protein, the nemesis of a "bland" diet, is supposed to encourage stomach acidity, though there is actually a high-protein diet (Muelengracht) that has been shown effectively to reduce it. Peptic ulcer has been called the "wound stripe of civilization," a phrase that emphasizes the psychosomatic aspect of the disease, and yet the antistress activity of properly used nutritional therapies has been ignored. A good example is found in pantothenic acid, known to be important to adrenal function, but less recognized for its effect in blocking the adverse action of cortisone on the stomach. Yet one of the well-known side reactions to cortisone drugs *is* stomach ulcer.

Pantothenic acid, vitamin E, and vitamin B complex, accompanied by a multiple vitamin-mineral supplement, have been used for stomach and duodenal ulcer, together with syrup of glycyrrhiza, which is licorice (not anise). Where possible, the supplements have been used in liquid rather than capsule or tablet form. The licorice must be used under medical direction, for it can cause side reactions, such as edema (swelling), which derive from a hormonelike effect. The combination proved so effective in the practice of a physician to whom I supplied these data that he remarked that he suspected cancer, rather than ulcer, when the therapy failed to promote healing. Higher dosages than those recommended on the label, particularly of pantothenic acid, are employed by medical nutritionists. Dosage of the glycyrrhiza will be supplied to physicians on request.

VARICOSE VEINS

Too many sufferers with varicosities wind up with surgery—stripping of the affected veins. This is symptomatic treatment, the worst type of medicine, for the process that initiated that pathology has not been interrupted.

Reread the discussion of constipation, starting on page 63. As unrelated as that topic seems, it isn't, for the pressure used by the constipated to induce bowel movement exerts enormous pressure on the circulation, particularly in the left leg, and the first step in relieving some of the distress of varicose veins and helping to avoid a new outburst is to arrive at bowel movement without stress.

Forty years ago, in research that has been ignored, varicose veins were found to be seven times as frequent in women, after pregnancy, whose diets were poor sources of vitamin C. The use of vitamin C, vitamin E, and bioflavonoids has brought relief to many sufferers with this common condition. This suggests, of course, that a history of good diet is the best protection against varicosities, but with that, a reasonable amount of exercise is needed. That is at least implicit in the use of support stockings to treat the condition, for they supply what poor muscle tone will not.

Supplemental dosage, as suggested on the labels, is the prophylactic amount of these nutrients, but the medical nutritionist may go far beyond these in therapy.

EPILOGUE

Considering that nutritionists must often struggle with the failures of modern medicine, any degree of success that they achieve is real accomplishment. What you are about to read, which I write by way of taking leave of you, is the story of a few such achievements. I am painfully aware that a few case histories do not carve in stone a lasting truth, but they do teach an important lesson: You never surrender, you never give up. The first history is that of a little boy, retarded, burdened with cerebral palsy (spastic), a cleft palate, and a harelip. What happened with him led to the second history, that of my own mother, who had a stroke. That in turn led to the third history, of a young man who attempted suicide by carbon monoxide poisoning and almost succeeded, his story told by his mother.

Years ago, at the University of Illinois, Professor Thomas Cureton experimented with a group of out-of-condition, middle-aged Americans, men who agreed to partake of a program of exercise, gaited to their needs and tolerances, plus the use of a supplement of wheat germ oil in which one of the natural constituents, octocosonal, had been concentrated. He reported that the program reversed the physiological age of the participants by a number of years. My attention was drawn to the paper because I had been fascinated by the effectiveness of wheat germ oil as a treatment for *amyotonia congenita,* a disorder of the newborn in which the muscles are without tone, so weak that the children can't move normally. I had wondered which of the many constituents of wheat germ oil was responsible for the effect, and Cureton's research identified it as octocosanol, which to the chemist is one of a number of long-chain, waxy alcohols natural to the oil. The question arose immediately: Would this factor be helpful in any of the nerve-muscle disorders for which medicine has few, if any, answers and little helpfulness? My question was partially answered at the Payne Whitney Muscular Dystrophy Clinic, where a researcher found this wheat germ oil fraction useful. In fact, it was for a while known by his name—the Milhorat fraction.

From the manufacturer who supplied the octocosanol-enriched wheat germ oil for this physician, I obtained a supply of the material, which by that time had been renamed the "neuromuscular fraction." Endless vistas of potential research beckoned, but it was a year before the opportunity came to give this nutritional concentrate a therapeutic trial. That appeared in a telephone call from the Massachusetts Bay State Training Center, concerning a six-year-old who was being fitted for a back brace, for deformity of the muscles caused by disuse. The child already wore two leg braces and walked painfully with the help of two crutches.

A few months later, after experience with a few more spastic children, I mentioned the research in a broadcast and received a call from the medical director of the national headquarters of the Cerebral Palsy Society. He subsequently met with me, examined the serial photographs of some of the children, read the letters from Danny's mother, and returned to Baltimore, where he announced that nutrition would in the future play an important role in the treatment of cerebral palsy. There is only one catch: That was twenty-five years ago, and he has never asked me exactly what Danny took.

During the course of the next twenty-five years, I watched the response of some 300 sufferers with multiple sclerosis to octocosanol treatment. This note will tell you why. It comes from an officer of a hospital, himself a victim of MS: "Please accept my apologies for a late reply, but it did take time to locate and acquire the octocosanol. One tablet b.i.d.p.c. [twice daily, after meals] has been taken for the past two weeks. After the first three days on this regimen, the tremors in my right hand were so reduced that I was able to use my right hand in eating. I have used my left hand to eat and to shave with for the past several years. Furthermore, my handwriting—particularly my signature—was much more stable, not showing the effect of ataxia" (difficulty in controlling the limbs).

In my correspondence with the patient, I had indicated my willingness to obtain a free supply of the nutrient octocosanol for a clinical trial in the hospital population of multiple sclerosis patients. His response is frustrating: ". . . with reference to your doing a large scale clinical study with M.S. using octocosanol supplied without charge, unfortunately, I must tell you that the neurologists are not in favor of a study or patients taking it individually." (I am compelled to remind you that those same neurologists have *no* treatment for MS).

The last paragraph emphasizes the resistance of the drug-oriented establishment to harmless nutritional therapy, even when drugs yield not one worthwhile benefit in the disease. My correspondent says: "At this point I happen to be the only one actively taking octocosanol, and I don't see any way of denting the armor. As you are well aware, the physicians' knowledge of nutrition, particularly vitamins, leaves something to be desired. I will keep you informed of my progress."

I offered the fruits of this research to the multiple sclerosis society decades ago. Their response was to answer inquiries with a form letter, reading: "Dr. Fredericks' M.S. nutritional therapy is valueless, and we have never tested it." The department wasn't named, but probably was the bureau of the non sequitur.

Multiple sclerosis therapy is discussed at length in this text, but I paused to cite the letter you have just read, one of hundreds in the same vein, so that you will better understand your difficulty in locating practitioners competent in nutrition therapy for the disorder. I must add the caution that octocosanol, like exclusion of allergenic foods, isn't a panacea for MS. About 25 percent of the patients show a recognizable benefit, and achieving that almost always takes months, rather than days. The treatment, apropos of the difficulty of obtaining nutritional therapies from orthodox physicians, should be medically supervised, not because it's dangerous but because we *must* educate physicians for the benefit of the patients they may later serve.

Brain injury presents the same view of medical lethargy or active opposition to the use of nutritional aids. A typical history is that of a young man who attempted suicide via carbon monoxide from an autombile exhaust. He was brought to the hospital in decerebrate rigidity (a guarantee of brain damage in severe degree). With the patient unconscious and on life support, the following are the evaluations of the numerous professionals who were consulted:

1. This (the coma) is the best you'll ever see him. (attending physician)
2. He might progress to sitting in a chair, with normal breathing but voluntarily able to do nothing. (attending neurologist)
3. I've never seen alpha (brain) waves come back. His alpha are gone. (California physician)
4. It's too soon to tell. (medical nutritionist)
5. Octocosanol won't help. He should have had hyperbaric oxygen immediately. There are no medical nutritionists who can work in that hospital. They don't permit it. (another medical nutritionist)
6. It doesn't necessarily mean anything if there are no alpha waves. (Pittsburg researcher)
7. Take him home. They'll just let him die. (well-known psychologist specializing in brain damage)

The mother's conclusion, after being exposed to the fact that doctors know very little about the brain, make incorrect predictions, and don't agree with each other: "I said to myself, in my son's case, if I can find some rational thing to do, I'll do it [but] I have to err on the side of life. Even though the possibility of a Karen Ann Quinlan type of situation exists, a person shouldn't be left to die because of that possibility. The only way to know what kind of recovery they can make is to give them every help you can."

As the pioneer in research with wheat germ oil concentrate, the family had consulted me, agreed to nutritional therapy, and engaged the services of a medical nutritionist. This made it necessary to remove the young man from the hospital. He was placed in a private apartment, with twenty-four-hour nursing care, and the nutritional program started, using not only octocosanol, but evening primrose oil (which helps in the manufacture of prostaglandin E_1 as well as L-glutamine, which stimulates the central nervous system, plus a copious intake of protein, vitamins, and minerals added to a balanced diet in liquid form, fed at first via a nasal tube. Three and a half weeks later, the mother reported: "One of the nurses was telling the other nurse a very funny story. My son suddenly burst out laughing. I didn't sleep much that night—to know that he understood language and had memory was just too exciting." It was still more exciting to me, because humor is based on incongruity, and appreciating congruity (reality) is a requisite.

Bringing the history forward some months, after physiotherapy had been added to the regimen, the following is the patient's status, again as reported by his mother: "His speech has begun to improve. He squeezes my hand, sometimes. I recently told him I had done something which wasn't too bright. He commented, 'Pretty dumb.' He responds to key words appropriately: The name 'Ronald' brought 'Reagan,' plus the names of a few recent presidents. The term 'Santa' brought 'Claus,' etc. He is getting more control over his arms. He responds to 'knock-knock' jokes appropriately. He is able to tell me what he had for dinner. He has to learn again much of what an infant learns, in maturing. I believe he will be able to speak clearly and well, but it remains to be seen what his memory and reasoning will be."

It was in the late 1950s that I visited Dr. Andrew Ivy, seeking from this great physiologist a possible explanation of the action of octocosanol in brain damage. He said: "Don't speculate on 'rewiring' of the brain by octocosanol. It might encourage it, but I don't think that's the action. Don't conjecture on stimulation of maturation of neuroblasts [immature nerve cells] into neurons [mature cells]. The action is too fast for that." I responded that this left only the last possibility, which the textbooks and my neurology professor agree is impossible: stimulation of repair of damaged nerve cells. Dr. Ivy's response: "The textbooks are wrong."

Some twenty years later, I used octocosanol, vitamin E, bioflavonoids, and vitamin C for my mother, who had suffered a stroke that left her with left-side paralysis, impairment of speech, an immobile lip on the left side, and drooping of the left eyelid. I returned her to the physician four months later with one residual symptom—still a slight drooping of the eyelid, but no trace of the other symptoms. The physician then applied the therapy to twelve consecutive stroke patients, with eleven successes. His comment summarizes the problem of making inroads into a type of medicine that is drug-oriented and infatuated with double-blind studies. "There are," he cautioned, "spontaneous recoveries after strokes—but don't stop what you're doing."

Common sense will tell you that nutritional therapy isn't the magical cure for all ills. But considering that medical nutritionists begin where orthodox medicine has failed, modern medical nutrition has an astonishingly good record. It lays no claim to panaceas, but owes no debt, either, to the power of faith and suggestion. Not for nothing did Alexis Carrel remark: "The physician of today will be the dietician of tomorrow—or the dietician will be the physician." I accept the fact that posterity will view today's medicine as we today look upon the bloodletters of the Middle Ages; that our healing professions will be criticized, not for their ignorance, which will be understandable, but for their pretensions—which will seem unforgivable. I think, though, that the medicine of tomorrow will be practiced by a team: the medical nutritionist, applying what has been learned from the biochemist, the microbiologist, and the enzymologist. The beginning is here.

As the preceding lines were written, I heard a radio report that Tony Conigliaro, a well-known ballplayer, had "miraculously" returned to consciousness, greeting his mother after having been in a coma, following brain damage from a heart attack, for four months. Actually, his physician had called me for the protocols of the use of octocosanol in this condition, which I supplied. The patient's father sent me his thanks, in a radio interview, though he was not sure that the credit, at least in part, should not be given to the power of prayer. By coincidence, I replied, another patient—the young man with brain damage from carbon monoxide—was also in a Boston hospital, where he had made a similar "miraculous recovery." I do not denigrate the power of prayer but am vitally concerned lest, with the media shouting the "miracle recovery" theme, brain-damaged patients and their families will continue to suffer from the effects of delay—the worst form of denial.

APPENDIX

Sources of Additional Information

For technical information on "no-nightshade" diet for arthritis:

Dr. Norman F. Childers
Horticultural Publications
3906 N.W. 31st Place
Gainesville, Florida 32601

Bio-ecological medicine and allergy are addressed by:

New England Foundation for Allergic and
   Environmental Diseases
3 Brush Street
Norwalk, Connecticut 06850
(203) 838–4706

and by:

The Institute for Bio-Ecologic Medicine
820 N.E. 63rd Street
Oklahoma City, Oklahoma 73105
(405) 840–4357
Medical Director: Dr. William H. Philpott

This institution is particularly recommended for management of allergy and maladaptive reactions in epilepsy and in autism.

Chelation as a substitute for bypass surgery, as a therapy for impaired circulation in atherosclerois, and for senility can be obtained from members of:

The Academy of Medical Preventics
8383 Wilshire Boulevard
Beverly Hills, California 90211
(213) 878–1234

Your physician, if interested in immune-augmentation therapy for cancer and immune system testing for susceptibility to cancer, can query:

Immuno-Augmentation Clinic
Rand Hospital
Freeport, Bahamas
(809) 352–7455

Note: Costs of tests and treatments, availability of medical insurance, and acceptance of Medicaid and Medicare should be discussed with the practitioner you choose.

· Some societies charge a small fee for their directories.
· Be sure to enclose a business-size, stamped, addressed envelope with your inquiry.
· Do not insist on being referred to a practitioner in your home neighborhood. While the number of medical and other nutrition practitioners is growing steadily, there are many occasions when the patient must travel for competent care of this kind.
· If the patient is hospitalized, it may be difficult, even if the local physician is cooperative, to arrange for an in-hospital consultation. Hospital rules are often arbitrary in excluding consultations and therapies involving modalities not in the mainstream—meaning drug treatment—of modern medicine. It is often necessary to arrange such consultations when the patient has left the hospital.
· Finally, remember that nutrition isn't a panacea or a source of overnight cures. Generally, a problem that has grown with the years will not be solved in a few weeks of corrected nutrition.
Technical information *for physicians* on combined nutritional and drug therapies for Down's syndrome:

Henry Turkel, M.D.
19145 W. Nine Mile Road
Southfield, Michigan 48075
(313) 357–5588

Dr. Turkel's text, *New Hope for the Mentally Retarded,* is available from:

US for DS
P.O. Box 64405
Los Angeles, California 90064

Orthomolecular medical societies

As a health professional's license indicates that the practitioner has exhibited professional competence, so does membership in professional societies. But just as practitioners, though licensed, may vary widely in degree of competence, so may similarly accredited members of professional organizations. In seeking practitioners of holistic medicine, medical nutrition, and preventive medicine, both you and the referring practitioner, if any, should have reasonable assurance that you will be cared for by a professional who is experienced in the management of problems like yours, and with whom you can have a good rapport.

The largest and best-known society with a national membership devoted to preventive medicine and nutrition and to nutritional prophylaxis and therapy is:

International Academy of Preventive Medicine
Suite 469
34 Corporate Woods, 10950 Grandview
Overland Park, Kansas 66210
(913) 648–8720

Also:

International Academy of Metabology
P.O. Box 15157
Las Cruces, New Mexico 88001
(505) 523–0513

The bulk of their membership is in California, but they may have members in your area, or within reasonable distance.

Another society with similar interests and distribution of membership is:

International College of Applied Nutrition
Box 376
La Habra, California 90631

Those interested in herpes therapy can query:

Dr. S. H. Sklar
647 Anderson Avenue
Cliffside Park, New Jersey 07010

If you are interested in children with learning problems, hyperactivity, autism, or hypoglycemia, guidance in orthomolecular medicine and nutrition can be obtained from

Dr. Bernard Rimland
Institute for Child Behavior Research
4756 Edgeware Road
San Diego, California 92116

and from

The New York Institute for Child Development
205 Lexington Avenue
New York, New York 10016
(212) 685-3630

It should be noted that there are orthomolecular psychiatrists who treat and some who specialize in problems of children with these problems. The Academy of Orthomolecular Psychiatry and other organizations listed below can supply referrals. For referral to physicians practicing chelation therapy:

Academy of Medical Preventics
8383 Wilshire Boulevard
Beverly hills, California 90211

For nuclear cardiography, to identify latent cardiovascular problems which are frequently missed in electrocardiograms:

Nuclear Procedures, Inc.
30 Hempstead Ave.
Rockville Center, New York 11570

Practitioners in Orthomolecular Psychiatry

For schizophrenia, depression, autism, hyperactivity, learning difficulties, senility, hypoglycemia, and cerebral allergies, contact the following:

The Huxley Institute for Biosocial Research
1114 First Avenue
New York, New York 10021
(212) 759-9554

Academy of Orthomolecular Psychiatry
1691 Northern Boulevard
Manhasset, Long Island, New York 11030

The Orthomolecular Society
2698 Pacific Avenue
San Francisco, California 94115
(415) 346-5692

Mental Patients Association
2146 Yew Street
Vancouver, British Columbia K6K 3G7, Canada

On Our Own
Box 7251
Station A
Toronto, Ontario M5W 1X9, Canada

Princeton Brain Bio Center
862 Route 518
Skillman, New Jersey 08558

Reference Reading

Orthomolecular Psychiatry Texts ☐ *The Food Connection* by David Sheinkin, M.D., and Michael Schachter, M.D. Indianapolis: Bobbs-Merrill, 1979. Cerebral allergy influence in behavior, emotions, and disease.

PsychoNutrition by Carlton Fredericks. New York: Grosset & Dunlap, 1976. Nutritional therapies in schizophrenia, depression, hyperactivity, autism, etc.

Diet, Crime, and Delinquency by Alexander Schauss, Parker House, 2340 Parker Street, Berkeley, Calif. 94704.

Food, Chemical, and Drug Allergies □ *How to Control Your Allergies* by Robert Forman. New York: Larchmont Books, 1979.

Very Basically Yours: An Allergy Cookbook by Human Ecology Study Group, c/o Bonnie Weidman, 5460 North Marmora Ave., Chicago, Ill. 60630.

Management of Complex Allergies by Natalie Golos, New England Foundation for Allergic and Environmental Diseases, 3 Brush Street, Norwalk, Conn. 06850

Modern Orthomolecular Nutrition □ Vitamin B$_6$
The Doctor's Report by John M. Ellis, M.D. New York: Harper & Row, 1981.

Dr. Carlton Fredericks' New and Complete Nutrition Handbook. International Institute of Natural Health Sciences, Inc., P.O. Box 5550, Huntington Beach, Calif, 92646, 1977 (3rd printing).

Mental and Elemental Nutrients: A Physician's Guide to Nutrition and Health Care by Dr. Carl C. Pfeiffer. New Canaan, Conn.: Keats Publishing, 1976.

Arthritis □ *The Nightshades and Health* by Norman F. Childers (see pages 12–13).

Arthritis: Don't Learn to Live with It by Carlton Fredericks. New York: Grosset & Dunlap, 1981.

Drugless Nutritional Therapies □ *Dr. Atkins' Nutrition Breakthrough* by Robert C. Atkins. New York: William Morrow & Co., Perigord Press, 1981.

Warning: Both your bookstore and your health food store carry many nutrition texts. Some of them, in both places, are unreliable. Some represent pure cultism. Some exaggerate the considerable potential of nutrition in prevention and treatment of disease. Some are well worth buying, reading, and remembering. Time and concentration will help you to separate the wheat from the chaff. You will learn to avoid texts that generalize, as if human beings had uniform reactions to foods and nutrients. Avoided should be those which generalize on personal experience: "Fish helped my multiple sclerosis; such a diet will help yours!" This will keep you away from the "one-note" nutrition "authorities," such as Nathan Pritikin. You will also, if wise, avoid those publications which consistently deride claims for avant-garde nutrition, or which dwell upon "4,000 cases of vitamin poisoning yearly"—a misstatement corrected by the FDA, but not by some propagandists masquerading as scientists. You should avoid those who view nutrition with alarm while silent on the dangers of drugs, food additives, surgery, and irradiation, such as Victor Herbert, Ronald Deutsch, Stephen Barrett, the American Council for Science and Health, Fredrick Stare, and other voices for the processed food industry.

INDEX

acetylcholine synthesis, 62
  and glaucoma, 62
  and mental retardation, 121
  and myasthenia gravis, 124
  and senility, 161
acne, 1
addiction
  allergic, 3, 155
  drug, therapy for, 50, 56-58
adenosine-5-monophosphate (My-B-
    Den), for herpes diseases, 31-32
adrenal cortex extract (ACE) for
    hypoglycemia, 103
adrenal function
  and diabetes, 38
  and hypoglycemia, 100, 102-03
  and pantothenic acid, 17
  in rheumatoid arthritis, 17
aging process and antioxidants, 7-8,
    129-30
  See also elderly, nutritional problems
    of; senility
alcohol intake and cholesterol, 88
alcoholism, 25, 56-58
allergies
  as addictions, 3, 155
  antihistaminic nutrients for, 50-51
  in arthritis, 18-19
  and body defenses, 5, 12
  cerebral, *see* cerebral allergy
  in cystic breast disease, 136-37
  in diabetics, 36-38
  and epilepsy, 60
  hay fever, 2
  and hypoglycemia, 6, 93, 94, 98, 110
  identification of, 2-5, 122

  injections for, 5
  and multiple sclerosis, 122
  non-food antigens, 3, 28
  rotation diet for, 6
  in schizophrenics, 51
  and shock therapy, 49
  small dose treatment of, 5
  symptoms of, 4-5, 12, 28
  vitamin therapy for, 6, 23
Aloe Vera juice
  for burns, 28
  for poison ivy, 156
aluminum toxicity, 163
  See also metal poisoning
Alzheimer's disease, 163
American Academy of Medical
    Preventics, 83f, 85
American Heart Association, 70
American Institute of Stress, 70
amino acids
  human nutritional needs for, 15
  sulfur-containing, as antioxidants, 7-8
  See also cystine; lysine; methionine;
    phenylalanine; tryptophane
amphetamines, use for hyperactivity, 92
angina, therapy for, 77, 81-82
ankylosing spondylitis, 24
anorexia nervosa, 147
antihistaminic action
  of calcium, 50
  of methionine, 50
  of vitamin C, 2
antioxidants
  and aging process, 7-8, 129-30
  for Crohn's disease, 35
  for neovascular eye disease, 62

burns, treatment of, 28
bursitis, vitamin B$_{12}$ for, 22

caffeine
  and alcoholism, 57
  and cystic breast disease, 135
  and hypoglycemia, 94, 99
calcium
  antihistaminic action of, 50
  and blood pressure, 74
  deficiency, and periodontal disease,
    152-53
  deposits in blood vessels, 84
    (See also atherosclerosis)
  deposits in joints, 13
  nutritional need for, 15, 161
  and osteoporosis, 142
  phosphorus-calcium ratio, 74
  sources of, 75
calcium pantothenate, see pantothenic
    acid
cancer
  bowel, 64-65
  breast, 130-31, 136, 139-40
  and cholesterol, 86
  lung, 21
  prostate, 156-57
canker sores, lysine for, 31
carbohydrate intake
  in diabetic diet, 36-37, 40
  optimal, 148
  and rheumatoid arthritis, 17
  for weight reduction, 147
carbon monoxide poisoning, 27
carotene
  conversion in diabetics, 37
  in peppers, 11-12
carpal tunnel syndrome, 29
carrot fiber for intestinal disorders, 67

cataracts, 62
  in diabetics, 39
celery, toxic constituents in, 9
cereals, allergy to, 18
cerebral allergy, 44, 49
  and epilepsy, 60-61
  and hyperactivity, 91
  vitamins for, 2, 92
cerebral palsy, therapy for, 27, 30, 121
cheeses, low-lactose, list of, 118
chelation
  for clogged blood vessels, 83-84, 162-
    63
  for metal poisoning, 83, 92
Cheraskin, (Dr.) Emanuel, 139, 147
Childers, (Dr.) Norman F., 12-13
chlorine, allergy to, 19, 46
chocolate, allergy to, 2
cholesterol levels in blood
  drugs to lower, 85-87
  body's need for, 87
  in diabetics, 37
  and heart disease, 69
  lipoproteins, 88
  low, and cancer, 86
  nutritional approach to reducing, 81-
    82
choline
  for diabetic neuropathies, 41
  in female nutrition, 134
  for glaucoma, 62
  for hypoglycemia, 110
  for memory improvement, 121
  for myasthenia gravis, 124-25
cholinergic crisis, 124
cholinesterase, 62
chromium glucose tolerance factor, 36,
    39, 126
circulatory problems in elderly, 158
    See also atherosclerosis

clofibrate, 8, 86
Coca, Arthur F., 2
colds
  allergic nature of, 2
  vitamins for, 23, 32-34
cold sores, therapy for, 31
colitis, 35, 67
  See also gastrointestinal disorders
collagen synthesis, 24
colon, disorders of, 64-67
  Crohn's disease, 34-35
compulsive behavior, *see* obsessive-
  compulsive behavior
constipation, 64-66
  and varicose veins, 166-67
cookbooks for nutritional guidance, 129
copper toxicity
  and depression, 44-45, 47
  and schizophrenia, 53
  symptoms of, 44-45, 47
  therapy for, 45
Cousins, Norman, 24
Crampton, (Dr.) C. Ward, 33
Crohn's disease, 34-35
cystine for epilepsy, 60
cytotoxic test for allergies, 19

degenerative diseases and nutrition,
  128-30
dehydration in elderly, 158
depression
  causes of, 5, 43-46
  schizophrenic, *see* schizophrenia
  therapy for, 45
diabetes, 35-42
  complications of, 39, 62, 88
  forms of, 36, 39
  mellitus, 39
  neuropathies of, 31
  and sugar intake, 75

tests for, 38, 100
  vitamin B for, 40-42
  weight factor in, 38
diarrhea as vitamin C side effect, 17, 23
Dilantin, use in schizophrenia, 50, 53
diuretics
  diet, 76
  drugs, 72-73, 160
  vitamin C, 62, 76, 157
diverticular disorders, 64-67
  and nightshade foods, 12
DMSO (dimethyl sulfoxide), 62
double-blind tests, 26
Down's syndrome, 119-20
  vitamin D toxicity in, 121
dreams, role of nutrition in
  recall of, 55
  nightmares, 42, 55-56
duodenal tissue for Crohn's disease, 35
drug addiction, therapy for, 50, 56-58
drug side effects
  and aging, 116, 159-60
  of anticholesterols, 86-87
  of antiepilepsies, 59-61
  of Beta-blockers, 77
  of cortisone, 166
  of hypertensives, 72
  of schizophrenia types, 43, 48, 50

ECT, *see* shock therapy
EDTA chelating agent, 83-84
eggplant, *see* nightshade plants
eggs
  antioxidant role of, 8, 88
  and heart disease, 88
  for rheumatoid arthritis, 16-18
  selenium source, 139
elderly, nutritional problems of, 158
  See also aging; senility
electrocardiogram (EKG), 67-68

Ellis, (Dr.) John, 29
emotional disorders, *see* nervous
    disorders
emotions and colds, 33
endometriosis, 133
enzymes
    and antioxidants, 8
    pancreatic, 8, 129
    supplements of, for elderly, 129
epilepsy, 59-61
    and allergies, 60
    Dilantin used for, 50
    manganese for, 48, 61
    as nutritional problem, 60-61
estrogen
    controlling activity of, 133-37, 140-42
    treating menopausal problems with,
        142, 143
evening primrose oil, 8, 25
    for arthritis and alcoholics, 25
    for Crohn's disease, 35
    for multiple sclerosis, 123-24
exercise
    eye, for myopia, 126
    and heart disease, 69-70
eyes, disorders of, 61-63
    cataracts, 39, 62
    exercise for, 125-26
    glaucoma, 62
    myopia, 125-26
    neovascular disease, 39, 62, 140
    retinopathies, 39, 63
    tear deficiency, 58

fast foods, sodium in, 79
fasting
    detoxifying effects of, 4
    to identify food allergies, 4
    of hospital patients, 126-27
fatigue, chronic, diet for, 149-50

fats and oils
    animal vs. vegetable, 89
    and blood cholesterol, *see*
        cholesterol levels in blood
    management of, in diabetics, 37
    and oxidants, 7
    partially hydrogenated, *see* trans fats
    polyunsaturated, 17, 149
    and prostaglandin E_1 synthesis, 58
Federation of American Societies for
        Experimental Biology, 81, 82
fiber in food
    deficiency, effects of, 64-65
    in carrots, 67
fish diet
    for multiple sclerosis, 122
    selenium in, 20-21
flatulence from bran, 66
flour processing, nutrient loss
        during, 64
folic acid
    for arthritis, 22
    for diabetic neuropathies, 41
    and estrogen activity, 135
    in schizophrenic diets, 50, 53
food additives, 120
    allergies to, 19
food aversion, *see* anorexia nervosa
food cravings
    allergic, 3
    pica, 155-56
food exchange lists for diabetics, 37
formaldehyde, allergy to, 19
Friedrich's ataxia, 81
fruits
    in diabetic diet, 40
    in multiple sclerosis diet, 123
    as source of bioflavonoids, 115
    as source of enzymes, 129

garlic for hypertension, 78

gastrointestinal disorders, 63-67

    Crohn's disease, 34-35

    of elderly, 128-30

    peptic ulcer, 165-66

gingivitis, vitamin B complex for, 28, 153

ginseng tea for menopause, 143

glandular therapy for adrenal failure, 103

glucose tolerance factor, *see* chromium glucose tolerance factor

glucose tolerance test, 38, 97-100

glutamic acid and brain function, 121

glycogen storage and Down's syndrome, 120

glycyrrhiza for peptic ulcer, 166

Goodheart, (Dr.) George, 4

Goodman, (Dr.) Herman, 94

gout, 112

    and heart disease, 88

grains

    allergy to, 18

    source of selenium, 139

    source of vitamin E, 140

    whole, in diabetic diet, 40

hair

    diagnostic analysis of, 100, 103, 121, 155, 156

    graying of, and nutrition, 130

hay fever, vitamins for, 2

heart disease, 67-91

    and aging, 8

    and atherosclerosis, *see* atherosclerosis

    diagnosis of, 67-69

    and hypertension, *see* hypertension

    and nightshade foods, 12

    nutritional formula for, 81-82

    and smoking, 69-70, 88

    and stress, 70-71

    vitamins for, 89-91

hemorrhoids, 57, 65

hepatitis, vitamin C for, 24, 33

Herbert, (Dr.) Victor, 23

hereditary factors in depression, 43, 47

herpes virus, therapy for, 31, 32

hesperidin, 78

histamine levels

    in drug and alcohol addicts, 48

    minerals to reduce, 50

    in schizophrenics, 45-47, 50-53

hives, 4

Hoffer, Abram, 46

hormones

    imbalances, and "female" problems, 132, 133, 137-38

    prostaglandins, *see* prostaglandins

Horrobin, (Dr.) David, 154

hospitalization, nutritional preparation for, 126-28

hydrocarbons, sensitivity to, 5, 7, 19, 44, 47

hydrochloric acid production, measurement of, 128

hyperactive children, 91-92

    and food additives, 74

    hypoglycemia in, 92, 93

hyperinsulinism, 100-01

    and Ménière's syndrome, 119

hypertension, 69, 72-80

    and aging, 8

    from copper toxicity, 45

    drugs used for, 72-73

    and sodium intake, 73-75, 78-80

    and sugar intake, 75-76

    therapy for, 76-77

hypoglycemia, 93-111

    with adrenal failure, 102-04

in alcoholics, 57
and allergies, 6, 110
and autism, 26
causes of, 94, 100
"cocktail" for, 110-11
depression from, 45, 47
diet for, 104-09, 122, 149
and diuretic drugs, 72
glucose tolerance test for, 38, 98-100
in hyperactive children, 91
and hyperinsulinism, 100-01
Ménière's syndrome, 119
in schizophrenics, 53
self test for, 94-96
and sugar consumption, 75
supplements for, 38-39, 110-12
symptoms of, 93, 97, 111
therapeutic diagnosis of, 101

IgE reaction, 2
ileitis, *see* Crohn's disease
immune system
    and allergies, 5, 12
    and polyunsaturated fat, 17
    in rheumatoid arthritis, 10, 17
    and vitamin C, 23-24, 32-33
Immunoglobulin E reaction, *see* IgE
    reaction
inflammation, evening primrose oil for,
    25
infertility, 112-16
injections vs. oral vitamins, 31
inositol
    for diabetic neuropathies, 41
    in female nutrition, 134
    for hypoglycemia, 110
    for nerve-muscle disorders, 30, 121
    tranquilizing effects of, 77, 117
insecticide, allergy to, 19
insomnia, 116-17

from copper toxicity, 45
of schizophrenics, 50
Institute of Bioecologic Medicine, 61
insulin
    and diuretic drugs 72
    overproduction, and hypoglycemia,
        94, 98, 100-01
    and prostaglandin B_1 synthesis, 58
    therapy for diabetes, 38, 39, 41
International Academy of Preventive
    Medicine, 30
    Tom Spies Memorial Lecture, 15
iodine in female diet, 138-39

joint pain from copper toxicity, 45

Kaufman, (Dr.) William, 9
    osteoarthritis therapy of, 13-15
ketogenic diet for epileptics, 61
ketosis, 149
kidney disease
    and aging, 8
    stones, 23
kidney function and use of chelation,
    84, 85
kinesiological method of identifying
    allergies, 4, 5, 122
Knapp, (Dr.) Arthur, 63
kryptopyrrole, 51-52

lactation, diet for, 114-16
lactose intolerance, 117-18
lead poisoning, therapy for, 83, 92, 156
lecithin
    for acne, 1
    action of, 82
    antioxidant role of, 7
    and blood cholesterol, 81-82
    and brain function, 147
    in elderly diet, 161
    in female diet, 143

pernicious anemia, 28
  vitamin B_{12} for, 22
peppers, and arthritis, 10, 11
Pfeiffer, (Dr.) Carl C., 50
phenylalanine for Parkinson's
    syndrome, 46-47, 150
Philpott, (Dr.) William, 26, 61, 136
phosphorous-calcium ratio in diet, 74,
    152-53
pica, 155-56
pituitary gland function
  in "constitutionally inadequate"
    women, 144-45
  deficient in criminals, 146
  and Down's syndrome, 120
plastic sensitivity, *see* hydrocarbons,
    sensitivity to
pneumonia, vitamin A for, 33
poison ivy, vitamin C for, 156
potassium
  depleted by diuretics, 72
  for osteoarthritis, 15
  salt-potassium ratio in diet, 74
  sources of, 72, 80

potato, and arthritis, 10, 11

pregnancy, complications of
  carpal tunnel syndrome, 29
  depression, 44
  diet for, 114-15
  distortions of taste and smell, 54
  eclampsia, 113
  morning sickness, 29, 115
  at over thirty, 135
  stretch marks, 116
  toxemia, 113
  varicose veins, 167
  zinc depletion, 54

preservatives in foods, 7

prickly heat, vitamin C for, 156

processed foods
  additives in, 75, 91
  sodium in, 74, 78-79
  trans fats in, 164-65
  white flour, 64, 91
Prometol, 123
prostaglandins
  for Crohn's disease, 35
  and evening primrose oil, 8, 35, 154
  deficiency, symptoms of, 164
  and insufficient tear flow, 58
  synthesis of, 154, 164
  for periodontal disease, 154
prostate enlargement, 156-57
protein
  acids, *see* amino acids
  deficiency of, in drug and alcohol
    addicts, 57
deficiency of, in elderly, 160
  in female nutrition, 134
  predigested, for allergies, 6
  and rheumatoid arthritis, 16-17
  in schizophrenic diet, 53
psoriasis, 157-58
psychiatry, orthomolecular approach to,
    42-43, 45
pulse rate and allergies, 3
pyridoxine, *see* vitamin B_6
pyrroluria, 51-52, 55

RAST (radioallergosorbent) test for
    allergies, 5, 19
retinopathies
  diabetic, 39, 62
  retinitis pigmentosa, 63
rheumatoid arthritis, 10, 16-18
  allergy in, 18-19
  therapy for, 18
riboflavin for periodontal disease, 153-
    154

Rimland, (Dr.) Bernard, 27
Rinkel test for food allergies, 5, 19, 122
Rosch, (Dr.) Paul, 70
Rinse, Jacobus, 82, 89
rotation diet for multiple food allergies,
    6, 19
"royal" jelly for rheumatoid arthritis, 17-
    18
rutin, 78

salt in diet, see sodium in diet
schizophrenia
    causes of, 45-48
    drug therapies for, 43, 48, 50
    and hypoglycemia, 53, 93
    high histamine type, 45-46, 50
    low histamine type, 52-53
    orthomolecular therapy for, 23, 42-43
    prevention of, 53-54
    pyrroluria, 51-52
    shock therapy for, 49
Schroeder, (Dr.) Henry, 64
scratch test for allergies, 5, 19
seafood allergies, 2
selenium
    anticancer role of, 139-40
    antioxidant role of, 7, 20
    for heart disease, 89-90
    for multiple sclerosis, 124
    for neovascular eye disorders, 62, 63
    for rheumatoid arthritis, 18, 20
Seligmann, (Dr.) Wolfgang, 40
Selye, (Dr.) Hans, 38
senility, causes and treatment of, 158-
    163
    See also elderly, nutritional problems
        of
serotonin levels in brain
    tranquilizing effects of, 47, 117
    and tryptophane, 47, 117, 147, 151

serum albumin levels in hospital
    patients, 127-28
shingles, therapy for, 31-32
shock therapy for schizophrenia, 49
shoulder-hand syndrome, see carpal
    tunnel syndrome
sinusitis, allergic, therapy for, 2
Shute, (Dr.) Wilfred, 34
Sjögren's syndrome, 58
Sklar, (Dr.) S. H., 32
smell, disturbances of, 54-55
Smith, (Dr.) Lendon, 121
smoking and heart disease, 69-70, 88
sodium in diet
    excess, excretion of, 100, 103
    in foods, 74, 78-89
    and heart disease, 72-75
    potassium-sodium ratio, 72, 74
    retention, and carbohydrate intake,
        149
sodium ascorbate, 23
solinase in nightshades, 11
Somogyi, Michael, 38
sorbitol, diabetic use of, 39
sphenopalatine block, 63
Spies, (Dr.) Tom, 14
    Memorial Lecture, 15
stress
    and allergies, 6
    and arthritis, 8
    and depression, 44
    and heart disease,70-71, 88
    and hypoglycemia, 94,102
    and multiple sclerosis, 122
stress adaptation syndrome, 38
strokes, brain damage from, 27
sublingual
    administration of medication and
        vitamins, 22, 129
    allergy tests, 5, 19